101 TIPS FOR A HEALTHY LIFE

Transform Your Routine into a Path to Well-Being

F. H. Rodrigues

ISBN-13: 9798324015466
ISBN-10: 1477123456

Cover design by: ADX Consulting and Digital Marketing
Library of Congress Control Number: 2018675309
Printed in the United States of America

*To all those who seek a path to wellness, may this book serve
as a guiding light on your journey to holistic well-being. May
it inspire you to nurture your body, mind, and spirit, and
may you find joy, peace, and fulfillment along the way.*

"Health is a state of complete harmony of the body, mind, and spirit. When one is free from physical disabilities and mental distractions, the gates of the soul open."

B.K.S. IYENGAR

FOREWORD

Embark on a transformative journey towards holistic well-being with our comprehensive guide. Packed with practical tips, insightful advice, and simple exercises, this book offers a holistic approach to nurturing your body, mind, and spirit. From cultivating mindful nutrition and finding inner peace to enhancing productivity and achieving quality sleep, each page serves as a roadmap to a healthier, happier life.

Key Features:
- Practical tips for cultivating a balanced lifestyle
- Insights on self-improvement and personal growth
- Guidance on mindful nutrition and healthy eating habits
- Techniques for finding inner peace and tranquility
- Strategies for enhancing productivity and achieving quality sleep

Join us on this journey to unlock your full potential and live a life filled with vitality, joy, and purpose.

PREFACE

In a world inundated with demands and distractions, the pursuit of holistic well-being has become not just a desire but a necessity. As we navigate the complexities of modern life, it's easy to lose sight of the interconnectedness of our physical, mental, and spiritual health. Yet, it is precisely this interconnectedness that forms the foundation of our overall well-being.

In this book, "A Journey to Holistic Well-being," we embark on a transformative exploration of what it means to truly thrive in every aspect of our lives. Drawing on ancient wisdom, modern science, and personal experience, we delve into practical strategies, insightful advice, and transformative practices designed to nurture not just our bodies, but our minds and spirits as well.

From the importance of mindful nutrition to the power of finding inner peace, each chapter offers a unique perspective and actionable steps to help you cultivate a life filled with vitality, joy, and purpose. Whether you're seeking to improve your physical health, enhance your mental well-being, or deepen your spiritual connection, this book is your comprehensive guide to holistic living.

As you journey through these pages, may you be inspired to embrace the fullness of your being and live each day with intention, gratitude, and authenticity. May you discover the profound joy that comes from aligning your actions with your values and honoring the interconnectedness of all life.

Welcome to the journey. May it be as transformative for you as it has been for us.

Warm regards,

F. H. RODRIGUES

F.H. RODRIGUES

101 TIPS FOR A HEALTHY LIFE

TRANSFORM YOUR ROUTINE INTO A PATH TO WELL-BEING

- Practical Tips for a Fuller and Balanced Life
- Discover the Secret to Lasting Health and Genuine Happiness
- Turn Small Changes into Big Results!

Are you ready to take the first step towards a healthier and happier life?

This book is your complete guide to achieving your well-being goals in a simple and practical way. With 101 carefully selected tips, you will discover how to make small changes that will have a big impact on your physical, mental, and emotional health.

Within this book, you will find:

- Nutrition tips to increase your energy and vitality.

- Simple exercises to strengthen your body and mind.

- Strategies to manage stress and cultivate inner peace.

- Advice to improve your sleep quality and increase your

productivity.

- And much more!

No matter what stage you're at in your wellness journey, start transforming your life today and discover the true meaning of lasting health and happiness.

NUTRITION

The secret begins with how we nourish ourselves. It's no secret that food industrialization has brought us various problems. Nutrition plays a fundamental role in our health and well-being. Each food we consume provides essential nutrients that our body needs to function properly and stay healthy. A balanced and nutritious diet not only gives us energy but also strengthens our immune system, improves cardiovascular health, promotes proper brain function, and helps prevent a range of chronic diseases.

If I could give you one piece of advice, it would be: Eat everything that has life. Everything you can plant in your backyard and flourish. Fruits, vegetables, greens. Remember: Everything that has life gives you life. Everything you eat that has undergone industrial processing takes away your life. The rule is quite simple. Now, let's see how Nutrition acts in our Body. We start our guide with valuable tips and an explanation for you to truly understand how everything works.

TIP 1: ENERGY SUPPLY

Carbohydrates play a crucial role in providing energy for the body. They are the main fuel source for the brain and muscles, helping to maintain energy levels and sustain daily activities. When we consume foods containing carbohydrates, such as bread, pasta, rice, fruits, and vegetables, these carbohydrates are broken down during digestion into smaller molecules of glucose.

Glucose is then absorbed into the blood and transported to the body's cells, where it is used as a source of energy for a variety of metabolic processes. The body's cells, especially those in the brain and muscles, rely on glucose to perform their normal functions.

For example, the brain uses glucose as its primary energy source to maintain cognitive function, concentration, and focus. Muscles use glucose to sustain muscle contractions during physical activities such as walking, running, or lifting weights. It is important to consume an adequate amount of carbohydrates in our diet to ensure that we have enough energy to meet the demands of daily life.

However, it is important to choose complex and whole carbohydrates, such as whole grains, legumes, and fruits, instead of refined carbohydrates, such as sugars and white flours, which can lead to rapid spikes and drops in blood glucose levels.

By balancing carbohydrate intake with other nutrient sources such as proteins, healthy fats, and fibers, we can maintain stable energy levels, promote satiety, and support overall optimal health.

TIP 2: TISSUE BUILDING AND REPAIR

Proteins play a vital role in the construction, development, and repair of the body's tissues. They are composed of amino acids, which are considered the "building blocks" of cells and tissues.

When we consume protein-rich foods such as meats, poultry, fish, eggs, dairy products, legumes, and nuts, our body breaks down these proteins into amino acids during the digestive process. These amino acids are then utilized by the body for a variety of functions, including tissue building and repair.

Tissue building and repair are continuous processes that occur in our body throughout life. For example, proteins are essential for muscle growth and maintenance of lean muscle mass. During physical exercise, muscles undergo microtears that need to be repaired and strengthened, and proteins play a crucial role in this recovery process. In addition to muscles, proteins are also critical for the health of bones, skin, hair, nails, and other body tissues. They help strengthen bones and joints, promote skin elasticity, and aid in cellular regeneration.

It is important to consume an adequate amount of protein in our diet to ensure that we have the necessary nutrients to maintain the health and integrity of the body's tissues. Individual protein needs may vary depending on weight, age, gender, level of physical activity, and health goals of each person.

By including a variety of protein sources in our diet, we can ensure that we are receiving all the essential amino acids needed to support the construction, development, and repair of the body's tissues, thereby promoting optimal health and overall well-being.

TIP 3: REGULATION OF BODY FUNCTIONS

Vitamins and minerals play vital roles in regulating a variety of essential bodily functions. They are known as micronutrients because they are required in small amounts but play significant roles in the body.

Vitamins:

Vitamins are organic compounds that perform a variety of functions in the body, from energy production to maintaining the health of bones, skin, and hair. They are classified into fat-soluble vitamins (soluble in fat), such as vitamins A, D, E, and K, and water-soluble vitamins (soluble in water), such as B-complex vitamins and vitamin C. Each vitamin plays specific roles in regulating bodily processes, such as hormone production, enzyme synthesis, and immune system function.

Minerals:

Minerals are inorganic elements found in nature and essential for human health. They perform a variety of functions in the body, including regulating fluid balance, maintaining the health of bones and teeth, transmitting nerve signals, and activating enzymes. Some of the most important minerals include calcium, iron, magnesium, potassium, zinc, and selenium.

A balanced and varied diet is essential to ensure adequate intake of vitamins and minerals. Nutrient-rich foods such as fruits, vegetables, whole grains, lean proteins, and dairy products are natural sources of vitamins and minerals essential for health. By consuming a variety of colorful and nutritious foods, we can ensure that we are getting all the micronutrients necessary to support proper regulation of bodily functions, thereby promoting optimal health and overall well-being.

TIP 4: PROTECTION AGAINST DISEASES

A diet rich in antioxidants, found in fruits, vegetables, and other whole foods, helps combat damage caused by free radicals and protects the body against chronic diseases such as cancer and cardiovascular diseases. A diet rich in antioxidants plays a crucial role in protecting the body against chronic diseases and strengthening the immune system. Antioxidants are compounds that help neutralize free radicals, unstable substances that can damage cells and contribute to the development of chronic diseases such as cancer, cardiovascular diseases, and neurodegenerative diseases.

Sources of Antioxidants:

Antioxidants are found in a variety of whole foods, especially in fruits, vegetables, nuts, seeds, and whole grains. Some of the best sources of antioxidants include berries (such as blueberries, strawberries, and raspberries), dark green leafy vegetables (such as spinach and kale), citrus fruits (such as oranges and lemons), nuts and seeds (such as almonds and chia seeds), and spices (such as turmeric and cinnamon).

Health Benefits:

Consuming a diet rich in antioxidants can help reduce the risk of chronic diseases, protect the body against cellular damage, and promote overall health. Antioxidants have anti-inflammatory properties and can help reduce inflammation in the body, which is associated with a variety of health conditions, including heart diseases, type 2 diabetes, and autoimmune diseases.

Tips for Including Antioxidants in Your Diet:

To increase your antioxidant intake, include a variety of colorful fruits and vegetables in your daily meals. Try adding berries to your morning cereal, making smoothies with fresh fruits and vegetables, and including colorful salads in your main meals. Additionally, aim to consume whole foods and minimally processed foods, avoiding foods high in sugar, trans fats, and artificial additives.

By making healthy food choices and including a variety of antioxidant-rich foods in your diet, you can strengthen your immune system, protect your body against chronic diseases, and promote optimal health and overall well-being.

TIP 5: THE ROLE OF NUTRITION IN PROMOTING HEALTH AND WELL-BEING

A balanced diet, consisting of a variety of nutritious foods, is essential for promoting physical, mental, and emotional health. By making healthy and mindful food choices, we can improve our quality of life and enjoy a full and vibrant life.

Nutrition plays a fundamental role in promoting physical, mental, and emotional health. A balanced diet, consisting of a variety of nutritious foods, provides the essential nutrients needed to keep the body functioning properly and promote overall well-being.

Physical Health:

A healthy and balanced diet provides the nutrients needed to sustain energy, promote proper growth and development, maintain a healthy weight, and prevent chronic diseases. A diet rich in fruits, vegetables, whole grains, lean proteins, and healthy fats provides the essential nutrients, vitamins, and minerals needed to maintain physical health.

Mental and Emotional Health:

In addition to affecting physical health, nutrition also plays an important role in mental and emotional health. Studies show that a healthy diet is associated with a lower risk of depression, anxiety, and other mental disorders. Nutrient-rich foods such as omega-3s, B vitamins, and antioxidants can help improve mood, reduce stress, and promote emotional well-being.

Quality of Life:

By making healthy and mindful food choices, we can improve our quality of life and enjoy a full and vibrant life. A balanced diet can help increase energy, improve concentration and focus, promote restful sleep, and strengthen the immune system. Additionally, a healthy diet can help reduce the risk of chronic diseases and increase longevity.

Promotion of Overall Well-being:

By adopting healthy and sustainable eating habits, we can promote overall well-being and achieve a healthy balance between body, mind, and spirit. A holistic approach to nutrition, which includes not only what we eat but also how we eat and how we take care of ourselves, can help us achieve optimal health and a full and vibrant life.

By recognizing the crucial role of nutrition in promoting health and well-being, we can make more mindful food choices and incorporate healthy habits into our daily lives, thus benefiting our long-term physical, mental, and emotional health.

TIP 6: MAKE SMART CHOICES AT THE GROCERY STORE

Prioritize fresh and unprocessed foods, such as fruits, vegetables, whole grains, lean proteins, and low-fat dairy products. Making smart choices at the grocery store is essential for maintaining a healthy and balanced diet. Here are some strategies to help you make more conscious and nutritious shopping choices:

Opt for fresh and unprocessed foods:

Whenever possible, choose fresh and unprocessed foods such as fruits, vegetables, whole grains, lean proteins, and low-fat dairy products. These foods are rich in essential nutrients and are generally healthier than processed and packaged foods.

Read food labels:

When choosing packaged foods, read the labels carefully. Check the ingredients and avoid products that contain artificial additives, trans fats, excess sugars, and sodium. Look for foods with simple and recognizable ingredients.

Be mindful of promotions:

While promotions can be tempting, they don't always represent the healthiest choices. Be mindful of offers on processed and packaged foods and opt for fresh and nutritious foods whenever possible.

Make a shopping list:

Before going to the supermarket, make a shopping list with the foods you need. This helps prevent impulse purchases and ensures that you only buy what is necessary for your planned meals.

Avoid shopping on an empty stomach:

Shopping on an empty stomach can lead to impulsive and unhealthy food choices. Shop after a meal or snack to help keep your food choices in check.

Try new foods:

Be open to trying new and varied foods. Explore different types of fruits, vegetables, whole grains, and proteins to add variety and nutrients to your diet.

By making smart choices at the supermarket, you can create a healthy and nutritious pantry that supports your health and well-being goals. Prioritize fresh, unprocessed, and nutritious foods whenever possible, and shop with mindfulness and intention.

DICA 7: PLANEJE SUAS REFEIÇÕES COM ANTECEDÊNCIA

Planning your meals in advance is an effective strategy for maintaining a healthy and balanced diet. Here are some advantages and tips to help you plan your meals effectively:

Advantages of meal planning:

- Saves time: Planning your meals in advance saves time at the grocery store and in the kitchen because you already know what ingredients you need and what meals you will prepare.

- Saves money: Meal planning helps reduce food waste and prevents impulse purchases, which can save money in the long run.

- Promotes healthy choices: By planning your meals, you have the opportunity to include a variety of nutritious foods in your diet and avoid unhealthy last-minute choices.

- Reduces stress: Having a defined meal plan provides a sense of control and reduces stress related to eating, allowing you to focus on other areas of life.

Tips for planning your meals in advance:

1. Set aside time for planning: Allocate time at the beginning of each week to plan your meals and snacks. Consider your food preferences, dietary restrictions, and busy schedules when creating your meal plan.

2. Make a shopping list: Based on your meal plan, make a shopping list with all the ingredients needed for your recipes. Be sure to check items you already have at home to avoid duplicate purchases.

3. Batch cook meals: Take advantage of free time to batch cook meals such as soups, stews, salads, and one-pot dishes. This makes healthy eating easier during the week, even on busy days.

4. Store food properly: Store prepared meals and fresh ingredients properly to ensure their freshness and quality. Use airtight containers to store food in the refrigerator or freezer and keep fruits and vegetables fresh in appropriate locations.

5. Flexibility is key: Be open to adjustments in your meal plan as needed. Things don't always go as planned, and that's okay. Be prepared to adapt your meals according to circumstances.

By planning your meals in advance, you can ensure that you

have healthy options readily available and make the process of healthy eating easier throughout the week. Take the time to plan your meals and enjoy the benefits of a more mindful and balanced diet.

TIP 8: READ FOOD LABELS

Familiarizing yourself with reading food labels is an important skill for making healthy and mindful food choices. Here are some guidelines to help you better understand food labels:

1. Ingredients:

- Check the ingredient list to understand which substances are present in the product. Ingredients are listed in order of quantity, with the most abundant ingredients appearing at the top of the list. Prioritize foods with simple and recognizable ingredients.

2. Nutritional Content:

- Look at the nutrition facts table to understand the nutritional content of the product. This includes information about calories, fats, carbohydrates, proteins, fibers, and other nutrients. Pay attention to serving sizes and the amounts of nutrients per serving.

3. Added Sugars:

- Check the amount of added sugars in the product. Avoid products with high levels of added sugars, as excessive sugar consumption is associated with various health issues, including obesity, diabetes, and heart diseases.

4. Saturated and Trans Fats:

- Limit the intake of saturated fats and trans fats, which can increase the risk of heart diseases and other health problems. Avoid products containing excessive saturated fats and trans fats.

5. Sodium:

- Reduce sodium intake, which is linked to high blood pressure and increased risk of heart diseases. Avoid products with high sodium content and opt for low-sodium versions whenever possible.

6. Artificial Additives:

- Avoid products containing artificial additives, colorings, flavorings, and preservatives. These ingredients may have long-term negative effects on health and provide no nutritional benefits.

By reading food labels, you can make more informed decisions about your diet and choose products that promote your health and well-being. Prioritize foods with natural ingredients, low levels of added sugar, saturated fats, and sodium, and avoid products with excessive artificial additives.

TIP 9: PRACTICE PORTION CONTROL

Practicing portion control is crucial for maintaining a balanced and healthy diet. Here are some tips to help you control your portions and maintain the proper balance between different food groups:

1. Know serving sizes:

   - Familiarize yourself with recommended serving sizes for different foods. Use standard measurements like cups, spoons, and a kitchen scale to ensure you're consuming appropriate portions.

2. Balance food groups:

   - Maintain the proper balance between different food groups in your meals. This includes foods rich in carbohydrates (such as whole grains), lean proteins (like lean meats, fish, eggs, and legumes), and healthy fats (such as avocados, nuts, and seeds).

3. Avoid overeating:

   - Avoid overeating, even of healthy foods. Practice moderation and pay attention to your feelings of hunger and satiety. Eat slowly, chew your food well, and stop eating when you're satisfied.

4. Use smaller plates:

- Use smaller plates to help control portions. Larger plates can lead to larger portions, while smaller plates can help reduce portion size and prevent overeating.

5. Plan your meals:

- Plan your meals in advance and divide your plate into sections to ensure a balanced distribution of foods. Reserve half the plate for vegetables, a quarter for proteins, and a quarter for carbohydrates.

6. Be mindful during meals:

- Be present and mindful during meals. Avoid distractions like television, cell phones, or computers, and focus on savoring and enjoying your food.

7. Practice self-discipline:

- Practice self-discipline and learn to say no to extra portions or unhealthy foods. Remember that portion control is an important part of a healthy and balanced diet.

By practicing portion control, you can ensure that you're consuming the right amount of food to meet your nutritional needs and maintain a healthy and balanced diet. Maintain balance between food groups, avoid overeating, and practice moderation in your daily food choices.

TIP 10: DON'T DEPRIVE YOURSELF OF FOODS YOU LOVE

It's important to remember that a healthy diet doesn't mean giving up the foods you love. Here are some tips to find balance between enjoying your favorite foods and maintaining a healthy diet:

1. Allow moderate indulgences:

- Enjoy your favorite foods occasionally, but in controlled portions. Allowing yourself moderate indulgences can help satisfy your cravings without compromising your health goals.

2. Practice balance:

- Find the right balance between healthy foods and indulgent foods in your diet. This means you can enjoy an occasional ice cream without feeling guilty, as long as you maintain a balanced diet overall.

3. Be mindful:

- Be mindful of your food choices and how often you consume indulgent foods. Make conscious choices and reserve special moments to enjoy your favorite foods.

4. Plan ahead:

- If you know you're going to have an indulgent meal on a certain day, plan ahead by making healthier choices for other meals. This helps balance your calorie intake throughout the day.

5. Savor every bite:

- When eating your favorite foods, savor every bite and appreciate the flavor and texture of the food. Mindful eating can help you feel more satisfied and reduce the desire for more.

6. Avoid guilt:

- Don't punish yourself for indulging in indulgent foods. Remember that moderation is key and that an occasional slip-up doesn't ruin your entire diet. Get back to your healthy routine at the next meal and move on.

By not depriving yourself of the foods you love and allowing moderate indulgences, you can maintain balance and satisfaction in your diet. Remember that a healthy diet is a journey, not a total restriction, and finding the right balance is key to long-term success.

The diet follows various patterns that society constantly tries to impose on our tables. Remember that what brings life, gives you life. What is disseminated is part of the social machinery to sell, not necessarily a nutritious food. Correctly follow these valuable tips and you will live an unprecedented transformation in all aspects of your life.

Aligned with nutrition, we continue our tips with Simple

Exercises to Strengthen Your Body and Mind.

Regular physical exercise not only strengthens the body but also has a significant positive impact on mental health. Exercise is a powerful tool for reducing stress, improving mood, increasing energy, and promoting an overall sense of well-being. Additionally, it strengthens muscles, improves flexibility and endurance, and helps maintain a healthy weight.

In this topic, we will present 20 simple exercises that can be done at home, in the park, or anywhere, without the need for special equipment. These exercises aim to strengthen the body and mind, providing a holistic approach to physical and mental well-being. From stretching and muscle-strengthening exercises to relaxation techniques and meditation, there are a variety of options for all fitness levels and personal preferences.

Ready to strengthen your body and mind in a simple and effective way? Let's explore these exercises together!

TIP 11: NECK STRETCH

Gently tilt your head to one side and hold for 15-30 seconds, then repeat on the other side. This exercise relieves tension in the neck and shoulders.

Neck stretching is a simple yet powerful practice that offers a range of benefits for the body and mind.

Benefits:

- Tension relief: This exercise helps relieve tension accumulated in the muscles of the neck and shoulders, especially after long periods of sedentary work or emotional tension.

- Improved flexibility: By gently tilting your head to the sides, you stretch the muscles of the neck, increasing flexibility and range of motion in that area.

- Discomfort reduction: Regular neck stretching can help reduce discomfort caused by muscle aches, stiffness, and tension in the cervical region.

- Mental relaxation: The gentle and mindful movement during neck stretching can help calm the mind, reduce stress, and promote an overall sense of relaxation and well-being.

Body Representation:

The neck is an area of the body that tends to accumulate a significant amount of tension due to poor posture, emotional stress, and repetitive activities such as using computers or cell phones. Neck stretching is an effective way to release this tension, improving blood circulation, increasing muscle flexibility, and relieving pressure on the cervical joints.

By gently tilting your head to the sides and holding the position, you stretch the muscles of the neck and shoulders, promoting relaxation and relief from stiffness. This exercise also stimulates the nerves and blood vessels of the cervical region, helping to reduce pain and improve neck mobility.

Regular practice of neck stretching not only relieves muscle tension and stiffness but also promotes a more upright posture, improves sleep quality, and contributes to an overall sense of physical and mental well-being.

TIP 12: PUSH-UPS

Start in a plank position and lower your body until your chest almost touches the ground. Push back up. This exercise strengthens the muscles of the chest, arms, and shoulders.

Let's explore the second exercise in detail:

Push-ups: Push-ups are a classic exercise that offers a range of benefits for strengthening the muscles of the chest, arms, and shoulders.

Benefits:

- Muscle strengthening: This exercise is highly effective for strengthening the chest, triceps, shoulders, and even core muscles when performed correctly.

- Stability development: Push-ups help develop stability and endurance in the core muscles, contributing to a stronger and healthier posture.

- Muscle definition improvement: By progressively challenging the muscles, push-ups can help increase muscle definition in the arms, chest, and shoulders.

- Increased resistance: Regularly practicing push-ups can increase muscle endurance, allowing you to perform other physical activities more easily and for longer periods.

Body Representation:

Push-ups are a highly functional exercise that recruits multiple muscle groups simultaneously. By starting in the plank position and bending your arms until your chest almost touches the ground, you are challenging the muscles of the chest, triceps, and shoulders to support and move the body weight in a controlled manner.

This movement not only strengthens the target muscles but also requires trunk stability, engaging the core muscles to maintain proper posture throughout the exercise.

As you perform push-ups regularly and increase the difficulty of the exercise, whether by increasing the number of repetitions or adding variations such as elevated push-ups or close-grip push-ups, you progressively challenge your muscles to promote growth and muscle definition.

Regularly practicing push-ups as part of a strength training program can lead to significant improvements in strength, endurance, and muscle definition, contributing to overall health and fitness.

TIP 13: SQUATS

Stand with your feet shoulder-width apart and squat down as if sitting in a chair, keeping your knees aligned with your ankles. This exercise strengthens the legs and glutes.

Squats are one of the most effective exercises for strengthening the legs and glutes, providing a range of benefits for the body.

Benefits:

- Leg strengthening: Squats work the quadriceps, hamstrings, and adductor muscles of the legs, strengthening these muscle groups comprehensively.

- Glute development: This exercise is highly effective for strengthening the glute muscles, helping to tone and define the gluteal region.

- Improved stability and balance: When performing squats, you challenge the stabilizing muscles of the legs and core, promoting greater stability and body balance.

- Increased mobility: Squats help improve the mobility of the hip, knee, and ankle joints, contributing to better range of motion and flexibility.

Body Representation:

Squats are a functional exercise that mimics the movement of sitting and standing up, involving a series of muscle groups to perform the movement effectively. By standing with your feet shoulder-width apart and squatting down as if sitting in a chair, you are recruiting the muscles of the legs, glutes, and core to support and move the body weight.

During the squat movement, it is important to keep the knees aligned with the ankles and prevent them from collapsing inward or outward to ensure even weight distribution and prevent injuries. Additionally, maintaining an upright posture and lifted chest helps protect the spine and promote good form throughout the exercise.

By regularly practicing squats and progressively increasing the difficulty of the exercise, whether by adding additional weight or performing variations such as jump squats or single-leg squats, you challenge your muscles to promote muscle growth and strength.

Incorporating squats into your strength training routine can lead to significant improvements in leg strength, core stability, and body balance, contributing to better athletic performance and a higher quality of life.

TIP 14: PLANK:

Keep your body straight like a plank, with your forearms on the floor and your toes on the ground. Hold the position for 30-60 seconds to strengthen the core and abdominal muscles.

Let's explore the fourth exercise in detail:

The plank is a highly effective static exercise that strengthens the core and abdominal muscles, providing a series of benefits for the body.

Benefits:

- Core strengthening: The plank is one of the best exercises for strengthening the core muscles, including the abdominal, obliques, lower back, and glutes, providing stability and support for the trunk.

- Improved posture: By strengthening the core muscles, the plank helps improve body posture, preventing back pain and injuries related to poor posture.

- Spinal stabilization: The plank helps stabilize the spine, promoting proper alignment of the spine during the execution of other exercises and daily activities.

- Development of endurance: Holding the plank position for an extended period challenges muscle endurance, helping to increase core strength and endurance over time.

Body Representation:

During the plank, you keep the body in a straight position like a plank, with your forearms on the floor and your toes on the ground. The elbows should be aligned with the shoulders, and the forearms parallel to each other. The body forms a straight line from the head to the heels, without letting the hips sag or rise.

This exercise challenges the core muscles and trunk stabilizer muscles to maintain the static position, which strengthens these muscles over time. It is important to keep the abdominal muscles engaged throughout the exercise to maximize the benefits and avoid unnecessary strain on the lower back.

By holding the plank position for 30-60 seconds, you challenge your muscle endurance and promote core development. Regularly practicing the plank as part of a strength training program can lead to a significant improvement in core stability, body posture, and muscle endurance.

TIP 15: DEEP BREATHING YOGA:

Sit in a comfortable position, close your eyes, and breathe deeply through your nose, inflating your abdomen and expanding your lungs. Exhale slowly through your mouth. This exercise helps calm the mind and reduce stress.

Let's detail the fifth exercise:

Deep Breathing Yoga is a simple and powerful practice that promotes mental calmness, reduces stress, and improves breathing quality.

Benefits:

- Stress reduction: Deep and conscious breathing helps calm the nervous system, reducing cortisol levels and promoting a sense of tranquility and relaxation.

- Increased body awareness: By focusing on breathing and body movement, you develop greater body awareness, promoting connection between mind and body.

- Improved respiratory function: Regular deep breathing

practice can improve lung capacity and respiratory efficiency, providing more effective and energizing breathing.

- Promotion of mental clarity: Conscious breathing helps calm the mind, reducing mental agitation and promoting greater clarity, focus, and concentration.

Body Representation:

To practice Deep Breathing Yoga, you can start by sitting in a comfortable position, with a straight back and closed eyes. Place your hands on your abdomen to feel the expansion and contraction of the body during breathing.

Inhale deeply through the nose, inflating the abdomen and expanding the lungs, allowing the air to fully fill the lungs. Then, exhale slowly through the mouth, releasing the air in a controlled and conscious manner.

Focus on the quality of your breath, trying to make it smooth, deep, and rhythmic. By practicing Deep Breathing Yoga, you may notice a sense of calm and relaxation spreading throughout the body as the mind quiets down and stress diminishes.

This practice can be done anytime and anywhere, whenever you feel the need to relax and recharge. Dedicate a few minutes of your day to practicing Deep Breathing Yoga and enjoy its numerous benefits for the body, mind, and spirit.

TIP 16: SIDE PLANK:

Lie on your side, supporting yourself on your forearm and feet, forming a straight line with your body. Hold the position for 30-60 seconds on each side to strengthen the obliques and core muscles.

The side plank is a variation of the traditional plank exercise that focuses on strengthening the oblique muscles and core muscles in a more specific way.

Benefits:

- Strengthening the oblique muscles: By supporting yourself on one forearm and your feet and maintaining a straight line with your body, you challenge the oblique muscles, located on the sides of the trunk, to sustain and stabilize the position.

- Core stabilization: Side plank is highly effective for strengthening the core muscles, including the deep abdominal muscles and muscles stabilizing the spine.

- Improved balance and posture: By performing the side plank, you develop greater body awareness and stability, promoting proper alignment of the spine and a more upright posture.

- Reduced risk of injuries: Strengthening the core muscles is essential for protecting the spine and preventing back injuries during physical activities and daily tasks.

Body Representation:

To practice the side plank, lie on your side, supporting yourself on one forearm and your feet, forming a straight line with your body. The elbow should be aligned with the shoulder and the forearm perpendicular to the body. Keep your body elevated from the ground, activating the core muscles to sustain the position.

By holding the side plank position for 30-60 seconds on each side, you effectively strengthen the oblique muscles and core muscles. Make sure to keep the breath flowing freely and avoid holding your breath during the exercise.

Side plank is a challenging but highly effective exercise for strengthening the core muscles and promoting trunk stability. Regularly practicing this exercise can lead to a significant improvement in core strength, stability, and endurance, contributing to better athletic performance and a lower risk of injuries.

TIP 17: HIGH KNEES:

Run in place, lifting your knees toward your chest. This exercise increases heart rate and improves cardiovascular endurance.

Let's detail the seventh exercise:

High knees are a simple and effective cardiovascular exercise that can be performed anywhere, without the need for specific equipment.

Benefits:

- Increased heart rate: High knees are an excellent way to quickly elevate heart rate, providing an effective cardiovascular workout.

- Improved cardiovascular endurance: By performing high knees for an extended period, you challenge the cardiovascular system, promoting greater endurance and aerobic capacity.

- Calorie burning: This exercise is a great option for burning calories and promoting weight loss, especially when combined with a healthy and balanced diet.

- Strengthening leg muscles: By lifting your knees toward your chest during high knees, you work the leg muscles, including the quadriceps, hamstrings, and calves.

Body Representation:

To practice high knees, simply run in place, lifting your knees toward your chest. Keep your arms moving as if you were running outdoors, and maintain a steady and vigorous pace.

While performing high knees, focus on maintaining good posture, with an upright torso and relaxed shoulders. Keep the abdomen engaged and breathe deeply to supply oxygen to the muscles and maintain energy during the exercise.

This exercise can be adapted to meet your needs and fitness level by increasing or decreasing intensity and duration as needed. Try different variations, such as running with higher knees or increasing speed, to challenge your body in new ways.

High knees are a convenient and effective way to improve cardiovascular health, increase endurance, and burn calories, making them a valuable addition to your exercise program.

TIP 18: LEG STRETCH:

Sit on the floor and extend one leg forward, reaching for your toes with your hands. Hold the position for 15-30 seconds and then switch legs. This exercise stretches the leg muscles and improves flexibility.

The leg stretch is a simple and effective exercise for stretching the leg muscles and improving flexibility.

Benefits:

- Improved flexibility: This exercise helps increase the flexibility of the leg muscles, including the hamstrings, quadriceps, calves, and muscles of the lower back.

- Muscle tension relief: Leg stretching helps relieve muscle tension and tightness, providing a sense of relaxation and well-being.

- Injury prevention: By keeping the leg muscles flexible and stretched, you reduce the risk of muscle injuries during physical activities and daily tasks.

- Posture improvement: Good leg stretching can help improve

body posture by aligning the spine and reducing tension in the back and hips.

Body Representation:

To perform the leg stretch, sit on the floor with your legs extended in front of you. Bend one leg and keep the other extended, with your toes pointing upward. Lean forward from the waist and reach for the toes of the extended leg with your hands.

Hold the position for 15-30 seconds, feeling the gentle stretch in the leg muscles. Breathe deeply and relax during the stretch. Then, switch legs and repeat the process.

During the stretch, avoid forcing your body beyond its limit and never bounce or jump while stretching, which can cause injuries. Keep the movements smooth and controlled, focusing on breathing and muscle relaxation.

Leg stretching can be incorporated into your exercise routine as part of the warm-up before a workout or as part of the cool-down after a workout. Regularly practicing leg stretching can help improve flexibility, reduce muscle stiffness, and promote greater freedom of movement in your daily activities.

TIP 19: INVERTED PUSH-UPS:

Stand with your back to a chair, place your hands on the seat, and move your feet away from your body. Bend your arms down until your elbows form a 90-degree angle, then push back up. This exercise strengthens the triceps and chest muscles.

Inverted push-ups are an effective exercise for strengthening the triceps and chest muscles, using your body weight as resistance.

Benefits:

- Triceps muscle strengthening: By performing inverted push-ups, you work the triceps muscles, located on the back of the arms, helping to tone and strengthen this area.

- Chest development: This exercise also works the chest muscles, especially the upper portion of the pectorals, helping to promote a more defined and toned appearance.

- Improved shoulder stability: By supporting your hands on a raised surface, such as a chair, you challenge the stability of the shoulders, helping to strengthen the stabilizing muscles around the shoulder joints.

- Increased functional strength: Inverted push-ups are a functional exercise that helps improve strength and the ability to perform everyday activities that involve pushing and lifting objects.

Body Representation:

To perform inverted push-ups, start with your back to a sturdy chair or bench. Place your hands on the chair seat, moving your feet away from your body and keeping your arms extended.

Bend your elbows and lower your body toward the chair, keeping your torso straight and aligned. Lower until your elbows form a 90-degree angle, then push back up, extending your arms completely.

As you perform the movement, focus on keeping the core engaged and the shoulders stable. Avoid arching your back or letting your hips sag during the exercise.

To increase intensity, you can raise your feet on a bench or elevated platform. To decrease intensity, you can keep your feet on the ground and your hands on a lower surface.

Inverted push-ups can be incorporated into your strength training workout as part of triceps and chest work, providing an effective way to strengthen these muscle groups without the need for specialized equipment.

TIP 20: PLANK WITH ARM RAISE

Get into a plank position and alternate raising one arm towards the ceiling, keeping the body stable. This exercise improves balance, stability, and strengthens the core muscles.

Let's detail the tenth exercise:

The plank with arm raise is an advanced variation of the traditional plank exercise, which further challenges the core muscles, stability, and balance.

Benefits:

- Core Strengthening: By performing the plank with arm raise, you recruit the core muscles, including the abdominals, obliques, and stabilizing muscles of the spine, to maintain stability during the movement.

- Improvement of Balance and Stability: Lifting one arm during the plank challenges the body's balance and stability, forcing the core muscles to work even harder to maintain the position.

- Development of Arm and Shoulder Strength: Alternately

raising the arms strengthens the muscles of the shoulders, arms, and upper body, providing additional toning to the upper limbs.

- Increased Body Awareness: By practicing the plank with arm raise, you develop greater body awareness, learning to control and coordinate the movements of the arms and core effectively.

Body Representation:

To perform the plank with arm raise, start in a plank position, supporting yourself on the forearms and toes, with the body forming a straight line from the shoulders to the heels.

From this position, alternate raising one arm towards the ceiling while keeping the body stable and avoiding hip sway. Keep the core muscles engaged and the hips leveled to prevent any rotation or misalignment of the body.

As you raise the arm, focus on keeping the shoulders square and avoiding body leaning to one side. Hold the position for a few seconds, then return the arm to the floor and repeat the movement with the other arm.

To increase intensity, you can try holding the position for longer or adding a pulse when lifting the arm. To decrease intensity, you can perform the exercise by supporting yourself on the knees instead of the feet.

The plank with arm raise is a challenging exercise that provides several benefits for the body, including core strengthening, improved balance and stability, and development of arm and shoulder strength. Regularly practice this exercise to achieve significant results in overall strength and fitness.

TIP 21: SEATED MEDITATION

Sit comfortably, close your eyes, and focus on your breath, observing thoughts without judgment. This exercise calms the mind, reduces stress, and enhances mental clarity.

Let's detail the eleventh exercise:

Seated meditation is a simple and powerful practice for calming the mind, reducing stress, and cultivating mental clarity.

Benefits:

- Mind Calming: By sitting comfortably and focusing on the breath, meditation helps calm the mind, reducing mental agitation and promoting a state of inner tranquility.

- Stress Reduction: Meditation is an effective tool for reducing stress and anxiety, providing a moment to pause, relax, and recharge.

- Improved Mental Clarity: By regularly practicing meditation, you develop greater mental clarity and concentration, enabling you to deal with the challenges of daily life more easily and insightfully.

- Cultivation of Mindfulness: Meditation helps develop mindfulness, the ability to be present in the moment without judgment, leading to greater awareness and appreciation of life.

Body Representation:

To practice seated meditation, find a quiet and comfortable place where you can sit without interruptions. Gently close your eyes and begin to focus on your breath, observing the sensations of the air entering and leaving your body.

As you breathe, observe the thoughts and feelings that arise in your mind without holding onto them or judging them. Let them pass like clouds in the sky, maintaining focus on the breath.

If the mind begins to wander, gently redirect your attention back to the breath, without self-criticism. Continue breathing deeply and observing the breathing patterns, allowing the mind to calm and quieten.

Regularly practice seated meditation, setting aside a few minutes of your day to connect with yourself and cultivate a calm and balanced mind.

TIP 22: MODIFIED PUSH-UPS:

Support your knees on the ground and perform push-ups with elevated feet. This exercise is an easier variation of traditional push-ups.

Modified push-ups are a more accessible variation of traditional push-ups, allowing you to strengthen the muscles of the chest, shoulders, and triceps with less intensity.

Benefits:

- Upper Body Muscle Strengthening: Modified push-ups help strengthen the muscles of the chest, shoulders, and triceps, providing additional toning and definition to the upper limbs.

- Improvement of Form and Technique: By supporting the knees on the ground during push-ups, you reduce resistance and facilitate movement, allowing you to focus on correct technique and avoid injuries.

- Accessible to All Fitness Levels: This exercise is suitable for people of all fitness levels, from beginners to those with strength or mobility limitations, offering a safe way to strengthen the muscles of the upper body.

- Progression to Traditional Push-Ups: Modified push-ups serve as a gradual progression to traditional push-ups, allowing you to build strength and technique before advancing to more challenging variations.

Body Representation:

To perform modified push-ups, start lying face down on the floor with knees bent and feet elevated. Place your hands on the floor, slightly wider than shoulder-width apart, with fingers pointing forward.

Press the palms of your hands into the floor and extend your arms, lifting your body off the floor until your arms are fully extended, maintaining a straight line from shoulders to knees. Lower your body back to the floor, bending your elbows and keeping your knees on the ground to aid stability.

Repeat the movement for several repetitions, focusing on maintaining good form and controlling the movement in all phases. Concentrate on keeping the core engaged and the shoulders aligned throughout the exercise.

Modified push-ups can be incorporated into your strength training as part of triceps, chest, and shoulder work, providing an effective way to strengthen the muscles of the upper body with less intensity.

TIP 23: LUNGES

Take a step forward with one leg and lower your body until both legs form 90-degree angles. Return to the starting position and repeat with the other leg. This exercise strengthens the legs and glutes.

The lunge is an effective exercise for strengthening the legs and glutes, providing additional toning and definition to the lower limbs.

Benefits:

- Leg Strengthening: Lunges work the muscles of the legs, including quadriceps, hamstrings, and calves, helping to strengthen and tone these muscle groups.

- Glute Development: This exercise also activates the glute muscles, helping to shape and tone the gluteal region for a more defined and firm appearance.

- Improvement of Balance and Stability: By performing lunges, you challenge the body's balance and stability, forcing the stabilizing muscles to work to maintain the position.

- Increased Range of Motion: Lunges help improve flexibility and range of motion in the hip and knee joints, which can help prevent injuries and improve performance in other physical activities.

Body Representation:

To perform lunges, start standing with feet hip-width apart. Take a step forward with one leg, bending both knees until they form 90-degree angles.

Keep the torso straight and aligned, with shoulders relaxed and core engaged to maintain stability. Ensure that the knee of the front leg does not extend beyond the line of the toes to prevent injuries.

Push the body back to the starting position, pressing through the heel of the front leg to return to the starting position. Repeat the movement with the other leg, alternating sides.

Continue alternating lunges for several repetitions, focusing on maintaining good form and controlling the movement in all phases. Concentrate on balance and stability throughout the exercise.

Lunges can be incorporated into your leg workout as part of quadriceps, hamstrings, and glutes work, providing an effective way to strengthen the lower limbs and improve overall body stability and balance.

TIP 24: BACK STRETCH

Lie on your back and bring your knees toward your chest, holding onto your legs with your hands. Hold the position for 15-30 seconds to stretch the lower back.

The back stretch is an effective way to relieve tension and discomfort in the lower back, promoting greater flexibility and mobility in this region.

Benefits:

- Relief of back tension: The back stretch helps to stretch and relax the muscles of the lower back, relieving tension and discomfort associated with sedentary postures or strenuous physical activities.

- Improvement of flexibility and mobility: By regularly practicing this exercise, you can increase the flexibility and mobility of the spine, facilitating smoother and more natural movements in daily life.

- Prevention of back injuries: The back stretch helps maintain the health and integrity of the spine, reducing the risk of injuries and chronic back pain.

- Promotion of relaxation and well-being: This exercise promotes a sense of relaxation and overall well-being, helping to relieve stress and tension accumulated throughout the day.

Body Representation:

To perform the back stretch, lie on your back on a comfortable surface, such as a mat or mattress. Bend your knees and bring them toward your chest, wrapping your arms around your legs to help bring them closer to your body.

Hold the position for 15-30 seconds, breathing deeply and relaxing the muscles of the back and hips. Focus on feeling a gentle and comfortable stretch in the lower back, avoiding any excessive pain or discomfort.

While holding the position, you can gently rock back and forth or from side to side to increase the stretch and mobility of the spine.

After the specified time, release your legs and slowly return to the starting position, extending your arms and legs completely on the floor.

Repeat the back stretch as needed to relieve tension and promote relaxation in the back.

TIP 25: INCLINE PUSH-UPS

Support your hands on a raised surface, such as a bench or a wall, and perform push-ups. This exercise is an easier variation of traditional push-ups.

Incline push-ups are a more accessible variation of traditional push-ups, allowing you to strengthen the muscles of the chest, shoulders, and triceps with less intensity.

Benefits:

- Strengthening of the upper body muscles: Incline push-ups work the muscles of the chest, shoulders, and triceps, providing additional toning and definition to the upper limbs.

- Improvement of form and technique: By supporting your hands on a raised surface, such as a bench or a wall, you reduce resistance and facilitate movement, allowing you to focus on correct technique and avoid injuries.

- Accessible to all fitness levels: This exercise is suitable for people of all fitness levels, from beginners to those with strength or mobility limitations, offering a safe way to strengthen the muscles of the upper body.

- Progression to traditional push-ups: Incline push-ups serve as a gradual progression to traditional push-ups, allowing you to build strength and technique before advancing to more challenging variations.

Body Representation:

To perform incline push-ups, find a raised surface such as a bench, a table, or a wall. Place your hands on the surface, slightly wider than shoulder-width apart, with fingers pointing forward.

Keep your body in a straight line from shoulders to heels, with arms extended and core muscles engaged to maintain stability. Bend your elbows and lower your body toward the surface, keeping your elbows close to your body.

Push your body back to the starting position, extending your arms completely and maintaining good form throughout the movement.

Repeat the movement for several repetitions, focusing on maintaining good form and controlling the movement in all phases. Concentrate on keeping the core engaged and the shoulders aligned throughout the exercise.

Incline push-ups can be incorporated into your strength training as part of triceps, chest, and shoulder work, providing an effective way to strengthen the muscles of the upper body with less intensity.

TIP 26: ABDOMINAL CRUNCHES

Lie on your back, bend your knees, and place your hands behind your head. Lift your shoulders off the floor, contracting the abdominal muscles, and then lower back down. This exercise strengthens the abdominal muscles.

Crunches are a fundamental exercise for strengthening the abdominal muscles, providing stability and support for the torso and improving overall body posture.

Benefits:

- Strengthening of the abdominal muscles: Crunches target the abdominal muscles, including the rectus abdominis, obliques, and transverse abdominis, providing additional toning and definition to the abdominal region.

- Trunk stabilization: By strengthening the core muscles, crunches help stabilize the torso and spine, reducing the risk of back injuries and improving overall body posture.

- Improvement of athletic performance: A strong and stable core is essential for the effective execution of athletic movements and daily activities, such as lifting heavy objects, running, and participating in sports.

- Reduction of injury risk: By strengthening the abdominal muscles, you improve the body's ability to absorb impact and distribute stress more effectively, reducing the risk of injuries during physical activities.

Body Representation:

To perform crunches, lie on your back on a comfortable surface, such as a mat or mattress. Bend your knees and place your feet on the floor, keeping your knees aligned with your hips.

Place your hands behind your head, with elbows pointing to the sides, and contract your abdominal muscles to lift your shoulders off the floor, keeping the lower back pressed against the floor.

Exhale as you lift your shoulders off the floor, focusing on contracting the abdominal muscles and avoiding pulling your neck with your hands. Hold the contraction for a second at the top of the movement.

Inhale as you slowly lower your shoulders back to the floor, maintaining control of the movement and avoiding dropping your body back to the floor.

Repeat the movement for several repetitions, focusing on maintaining good form and controlling the movement in all phases. Concentrate on keeping the abdominal muscles contracted and avoiding excessive body sway during the exercise.

Crunches can be incorporated into your strength training as part of core work, providing an effective way to strengthen the abdominal muscles and improve trunk stability and support.

TIP 27: SPINAL TWIST

Sit with your legs extended in front of you, cross one leg over the other, and twist your torso in the direction of the crossed leg. Hold the position for 15-30 seconds, then switch sides. This exercise stretches the spine and back muscles.

The spinal twist is a stretching exercise that helps increase the flexibility of the spine and back muscles, providing relief from tension and stiffness.

Benefits:

- Spine elongation: The spinal twist helps elongate and mobilize the vertebrae of the spine, promoting greater range of motion and flexibility in the region.

- Relief of back tension: This exercise helps relieve tension and discomfort in the back, especially after prolonged periods of sitting or standing.

- Posture improvement: By stretching the back muscles and promoting greater mobility in the spine, the spinal twist can help improve posture and align the spine more properly.

- Mind and body relaxation: Performing this exercise can promote a sense of relaxation and well-being, helping to reduce stress and tension accumulated throughout the day.

Body Representation:

To perform the spinal twist, sit on the floor with your legs extended in front of you. Cross one leg over the other, placing the foot of the crossed leg on the floor next to the opposite knee.

Keep your spine upright and arms extended along the body. Then, twist your torso in the direction of the crossed leg, placing the opposite hand to the crossed knee on the floor behind you to help stabilize the position.

Hold the position for 15-30 seconds, breathing deeply and feeling the stretch along the spine and back muscles. Focus on maintaining an upright posture and avoid leaning backward or forward during the exercise.

After the specified time, slowly return to the starting position and repeat the movement on the other side, crossing the other leg over the first and twisting the torso in the opposite direction.

Repeat the spinal twist a few times on each side, focusing on gently and controlled stretching and mobilizing the spine.

TIP 28: WALL PUSH-UPS

Stand facing the wall, with arms extended and hands placed on the wall. Bend your arms and bring your chest towards the wall, then push back up. This exercise is an easier variation of traditional push-ups.

Wall push-ups are a gentler variation of traditional push-ups, providing an accessible way to strengthen the muscles of the chest, shoulders, and triceps.

Benefits:

- Strengthening of the upper body muscles: Wall push-ups target the same muscles as traditional push-ups, including the chest, shoulders, and triceps, providing additional toning and definition to the upper body.

- Reduced intensity: By placing your hands on the wall, you reduce the amount of body weight supported during the movement, making the exercise more accessible for beginners or individuals with strength or mobility limitations.

- Learning correct technique: This exercise allows you to become familiar with the correct technique of push-ups, including hand placement, range of motion, and proper breathing, before progressing to more challenging variations.

- Gradual progression: Wall push-ups serve as a gradual progression to traditional floor push-ups, allowing you to develop strength and confidence gradually as you advance to more advanced exercises.

Body Representation:

To perform wall push-ups, stand facing the wall at a comfortable distance, with arms extended and hands placed on the wall slightly wider than shoulder-width apart.

Keep your body in a straight line from shoulders to heels, with feet shoulder-width apart to provide stability. Keep elbows slightly bent and aligned with the shoulders.

Bend your arms and bring your chest towards the wall, keeping the body aligned and the core muscles engaged. Avoid letting the elbows flare out to the sides or the shoulders shrug towards the ears.

Push back up until your arms are fully extended again, maintaining good form throughout the movement.

Repeat the movement for several repetitions, focusing on maintaining good form and controlling the movement in all phases. Concentrate on keeping the core muscles engaged and avoiding arching the back or shrugging the shoulders during the exercise.

Wall push-ups can be incorporated into your strength training as part of triceps, chest, and shoulder work, providing an effective way to strengthen the upper body muscles with lower intensity.

TIP 29:
WARRIOR POSE
(VIRABHADRASANA)

Stand with your feet hip-width apart, turn one foot out, and bend the knee, keeping the other foot facing forward. Extend your arms to the sides and look forward. This exercise strengthens the legs and arms and improves balance.

The Warrior pose, or Virabhadrasana in Sanskrit, is a powerful posture that strengthens the legs, arms, and core while promoting balance and stability.

Benefits:

- Leg strengthening: The Warrior pose involves bending one knee while keeping the opposite leg extended, which strengthens the muscles of the legs, including quadriceps, hamstrings, and calves.

- Arm strengthening: Extending the arms to the sides, keeping them parallel to the ground, helps strengthen the muscles of the shoulders, arms, and core.

- Improvement of balance: The Warrior pose challenges balance and stability, encouraging concentration and body awareness.

- Stimulation of blood circulation: By engaging the muscles of the legs and arms, the Warrior pose increases blood flow to these areas, promoting cardiovascular health and transporting nutrients and oxygen to the muscle tissues.

Body Representation:

To perform the Warrior pose, start by standing with your feet hip-width apart. Turn one foot out so that the big toe points in the opposite direction of the body, and keep the other foot facing forward.

Bend the knee of the foot facing outward, forming a 90-degree angle, while keeping the opposite leg extended and aligned with the torso. Make sure the bent knee is aligned with the ankle to protect the joint.

Extend your arms to the sides, keeping them parallel to the ground, and look forward towards the horizon. Keep the shoulders relaxed and the core engaged to maintain stability.

Hold the Warrior pose for 30 seconds to 1 minute, breathing deeply and focusing on posture and breath. Then, repeat on the other side, reversing the position of the feet and bending the other knee.

Focus on maintaining good form and alignment during the Warrior pose, keeping the muscles engaged and the breath fluid.

TIP 30: PROGRESSIVE MUSCLE RELAXATION

Sit or lie down comfortably and tense and relax the muscles of each part of the body, starting from the feet and moving up to the head. This exercise relieves muscle tension and promotes deep relaxation.

Let's detail the twentieth exercise:

Progressive muscle relaxation is an effective technique for relieving muscle tension and promoting a deep state of physical and mental relaxation.

Benefits:

- Muscle tension relief: By alternating between contracting and relaxing the muscles of different parts of the body, you can release accumulated tension and promote a feeling of relaxation and well-being.

- Reduction of stress and anxiety: Progressive muscle relaxation helps calm the mind and body, reducing levels of stress and anxiety and promoting a sense of calm and tranquility.

- Improvement in sleep quality: Practicing this technique before bedtime can help prepare the body and mind for a more peaceful and restful sleep, promoting better sleep quality.

- Increased body awareness: By focusing attention on each part of the body during the exercise, you increase your body awareness and develop a greater ability to detect and release muscle tension.

Body Representation:

To practice progressive muscle relaxation, find a quiet and comfortable place to sit or lie down. Close your eyes and begin to breathe deeply, focusing on the sensation of breath entering and leaving the body.

Start with the feet and focus on tensing the muscles of the feet and toes for a few seconds, then completely relax the muscles, releasing any tension or tightness.

Continue moving up the body, alternating between contracting and relaxing the muscles of each part, including the legs, glutes, abdomen, chest, arms, hands, shoulders, neck, face, and scalp.

When tensing each muscle group, hold the contraction for a few seconds and then completely relax, releasing any accumulated tension. Feel the sensation of relaxation and lightness as the muscles loosen and relax.

Continue this process until you have gone through the entire body, taking as much time as you need in each area to experience maximum relaxation. At the end, remain lying down or sitting for a few moments, enjoying the feeling of deep relaxation and calm that accompanies this practice.

In these exercise tips, we have delved into a universe of possibilities to promote a healthy and happy life. From practical nutrition tips to a variety of simple exercises, our goal has been to provide readers with accessible and effective tools to transform their routine into a path to well-being.

We began by exploring the importance of nutrition as a fundamental basis for a healthy life. By understanding how food affects our body and mind, readers are empowered to make conscious choices that promote health and vitality. We explored how nutrients provide energy, aid in tissue building and repair, regulate bodily functions, and protect against diseases, highlighting the importance of a balanced and varied diet.

Next, we delved into the world of simple exercises, designed to strengthen not only the body but also the mind. From revitalizing stretches to yoga poses that promote balance and flexibility, each exercise was selected to offer tangible benefits for physical and emotional health. Progressive muscle relaxation, for example, not only relieves physical tension but also calms the mind, providing a refuge of tranquility amidst the busyness of daily life.

Our approach has been holistic, recognizing the interconnection between body and mind and emphasizing the importance of caring for both. By adopting a balanced approach that integrates nutrition, exercise, and relaxation, readers are empowered to cultivate a lifestyle that promotes lasting health, happiness, and well-being.

As we move on to the next valuable tips, we invite our readers to continue their journey towards a healthier and happier life, exploring new strategies and discovering the transformative power of small changes in their daily routine. Together, we can build a future of health and happiness, where each day is an opportunity to become the best version of ourselves.

Our journey towards a healthy and happy life is just beginning. We are ready to explore even more possibilities to promote physical, mental, and emotional well-being. We seek not only to provide information but also to inspire and motivate our readers to take action. Each practical nutrition tip and every simple exercise has been carefully selected to offer tangible and achievable benefits. We want our readers to feel empowered to take the first steps towards a healthier and happier life, knowing that they have the knowledge and tools necessary to do so.

However, we recognize that the journey to well-being is not linear and that each person will face their own challenges and obstacles along the way. That is why we are committed to providing ongoing support and guidance, so that our readers feel supported on their journey.

As we prepare to explore new topics and strategies in the upcoming chapters, we invite our readers to join us with open minds and open hearts. Together, we can learn, grow, and inspire each other as we navigate this exciting path towards a healthier, happier, and more meaningful life.

Strategies for Managing Stress and Cultivating Inner Peace

As we delve into the next chapter of tips, we embark on a journey toward emotional balance and inner serenity. In a world where stress seems to be a constant, it is essential for us to learn the art of managing our emotions and cultivating inner peace. This chapter is an invitation to explore a series of strategies and techniques that will help us face life's challenges with calmness, clarity, and resilience.

Our days are often filled with a myriad of demands and pressures, both personal and professional. Stress can manifest in various ways, affecting our physical, mental, and emotional health. However, by understanding the roots of stress and learning effective ways to deal with it, we can transform our experiences and find a renewed sense of balance and well-being.

Throughout this chapter, we will delve deep into the world of stress management, exploring relaxation techniques, meditation, mindful breathing, and much more. We will discover how to cultivate inner peace even in the most challenging situations and how to build a solid foundation for a quieter and more meaningful life.

What is Stress?

Stress is a natural response of the body to challenging or threatening situations. It is a physical and emotional reaction that occurs when we encounter demands that exceed our resources and coping abilities. Although stress is an inevitable part of life, when experienced in excess or for long periods, it can have significant negative effects on our health and well-being.

Stress can manifest in various forms, including physical symptoms such as headaches, muscle tension, and gastrointestinal problems, as well as emotional symptoms such as anxiety, irritability, and depression. Furthermore, chronic stress has been associated with a range of health conditions, including heart disease, diabetes, sleep disorders, and compromised immune function.

It is important to recognize that stress is not only a response to negative or challenging events. Positive situations, such as marriage, job changes, or the birth of a child, can also trigger a stress response. What matters is how we deal with these situations and how we can develop effective coping skills to manage stress in a healthy way.

TIP 31: PRACTICE GRATITUDE

Set aside a few minutes every day to reflect on the things you are grateful for. Keeping a gratitude journal can help shift focus to the positive in your life. Practicing gratitude is a powerful tool for cultivating inner peace and promoting emotional well-being. By taking a few minutes every day to reflect on the things we are grateful for, we can shift our focus to the positive in our lives and recognize the blessings and good things surrounding us.

Benefits of Practicing Gratitude:

- Promotes Emotional Well-being: By cultivating a mindset of gratitude, we can increase our levels of happiness and life satisfaction.

- Reduces Stress and Anxiety: Gratitude can help reduce levels of stress and anxiety, allowing us to focus on the present and the good things happening in our lives.

- Strengthens Relationships: Expressing gratitude to others can strengthen relationships and create a sense of connection and intimacy.

How to Practice Gratitude:

1. Keep a Gratitude Journal: Set aside a few minutes every morning or before bed to write down three things you are grateful for. This can include small things, like the sun shining or a meaningful conversation with a friend.

2. Express Gratitude to Others: Don't hesitate to express your gratitude to people in your life. A simple "thank you" can make a big difference in someone's day.

3. Practice Gratitude in Challenging Moments: Even in difficult times, look for something to be grateful for. This can help shift your perspective and find hope and comfort amidst hardships.

Practicing gratitude doesn't require grand gestures or efforts, but rather a mindset shift and a willingness to recognize and appreciate the blessings that are present in our lives every day. By incorporating gratitude into our daily routine, we can cultivate a deeper sense of inner peace and contentment.

TIP 32: DAILY MEDITATION

Dedicate a few minutes every morning to practice meditation. Meditation can calm the mind, reduce stress, and promote a sense of inner peace. Meditation is an ancient practice that has been used for centuries to promote mental tranquility, reduce stress, and cultivate a sense of inner peace.

By dedicating a few minutes every morning to meditation, we can reap a host of benefits for the body, mind, and spirit.

Benefits of Daily Meditation:

- Calms the Mind: Meditation helps calm racing thoughts and restless minds, providing a sense of calm and mental clarity.

- Reduces Stress: Regular meditation practice can help reduce cortisol levels, the stress hormone, in the body, leading to a sense of relaxation and well-being.

- Promotes Mindfulness: Meditation promotes mindfulness, or the ability to be present in the moment without judgment or distraction. This can help improve attention and concentration.

How to Practice Daily Meditation:

1. Find a Quiet Place: Choose a quiet and peaceful location where you can sit comfortably without being interrupted.

2. Assume a Comfortable Posture: Sit in a comfortable position with a straight spine and relaxed shoulders. You can choose to sit in a chair or on the floor with crossed legs.

3. Focus on Breathing: Gently close your eyes and begin to focus your attention on your breath. Feel the air entering and leaving your body, without trying to control the breath.

4. Let Thoughts Pass: As you meditate, it's natural for thoughts to arise in your mind. Don't worry about these thoughts or try to suppress them. Instead, simply observe them passing by, like clouds in the sky.

5. Return to Breathing: Whenever you find yourself lost in thoughts, gently bring your attention back to your breath. Use the breath as an anchor to the present moment.

6. Practice Gratitude: At the end of your meditation, take a moment to reflect on the things you are grateful for in your life. This can help end your practice on a positive note.

By incorporating meditation into your daily routine, you can enjoy a host of benefits for mental and emotional health. With just a few minutes of daily practice, you can cultivate a deeper sense of inner peace and well-being in your life.

TIP 33: CONSCIOUS BREATHING

Conscious Breathing: Practice conscious breathing in moments of stress. Focus on inhaling and exhaling deeply, bringing your attention back to the present moment. Conscious breathing is a simple yet powerful practice that can be used in moments of stress to calm the mind and promote a sense of inner peace.

By focusing on the breath and bringing our attention back to the present moment, we can reduce anxiety and cultivate a state of relaxation and tranquility.

Benefits of Conscious Breathing:

- Stress Reduction: Conscious breathing activates the parasympathetic nervous system, responsible for calming the body and mind, reducing cortisol levels, and other stress hormones.

- Promotion of Mental Clarity: By focusing on the breath, we can interrupt the cycle of negative thoughts and worries, promoting greater mental clarity and focus.

- Improvement of Respiratory Health: Practicing conscious

breathing regularly can strengthen respiratory muscles and improve the efficiency of the respiratory system.

How to Practice Conscious Breathing:

1. Find a Quiet Place: Seek out a calm and quiet environment where you can sit comfortably without being interrupted.

2. Assume a Comfortable Posture: Sit in a relaxed position, with a straight spine and relaxed shoulders. You can choose to sit in a chair or on the floor with crossed legs.

3. Close Your Eyes Gently: Close your eyes gently to reduce external distractions and direct your attention inward.

4. Focus on the Breath: Begin to pay attention to your breath, observing the natural movement of air entering and leaving your body. Don't try to control the breath, just observe it.

5. Inhale and Exhale Deeply: As you breathe, try to inhale and exhale deeply, filling your lungs with air and releasing it slowly. Focus on the rhythm and sensation of the breath.

6. Bring Your Attention Back to the Present Moment: If your mind starts to wander to thoughts or worries, gently bring your attention back to the breath. Use the breath as an anchor to the present moment.

Practicing conscious breathing regularly, even if just for a few minutes each day, can bring a host of benefits for mental and emotional health. By incorporating this simple practice into your daily life, you can cultivate a deeper sense of inner peace and well-being.

TIP 34: REGULAR EXERCISE

Engage in regular physical exercise to release endorphins, which are neurotransmitters that promote feelings of happiness and well-being. Engaging in regular physical exercise is one of the best ways to promote both physical and mental health.

When we exercise, our body releases endorphins, neurotransmitters known as "happiness hormones," which can elevate our mood and promote an overall sense of well-being.

Benefits of Regular Exercise:

- Release of Endorphins: During exercise, our body releases endorphins, which are chemicals that act as natural painkillers, reducing the perception of pain and promoting feelings of euphoria and pleasure.

- Reduction of Stress and Anxiety: Regular exercise can help reduce levels of stress and anxiety by providing a healthy outlet to release accumulated tension in the body and mind.

- Improvement of Mental Health: Studies have shown that

regular exercise can help reduce symptoms of depression and improve overall mood by increasing self-esteem and a sense of accomplishment.

How to Incorporate Exercise into Your Routine:

1. Choose an Activity You Enjoy: Find a physical activity that you genuinely enjoy, whether it's walking, running, swimming, dancing, practicing yoga, or lifting weights. Doing something you enjoy will make it easier to maintain a regular exercise routine.

2. Set Realistic Goals: Set achievable and progressive goals for yourself. Start with small goals and gradually increase as your physical fitness improves.

3. Schedule Your Exercise: Set aside specific time in your schedule to exercise, just as you would with any other important activity. Make exercise a priority in your daily life.

4. Vary Your Routine: Keep your exercise routine interesting and challenging by alternating between different types of activities and workout intensities.

5. Get Involved with Others: Consider exercising in groups or with a friend to add a social dimension to your exercise routine and stay motivated.

By making exercise a regular part of your life, you can reap a host of benefits for both physical and mental health. Remember that any amount of physical activity is better than none, so start today, even if it's just with a short walk or a few minutes of stretching.

TIP 35: TIME IN NATURE

Allocate some time to spend outdoors and connect with nature. Nature has a calming and restorative effect on the mind and body. Spending time outdoors and connecting with nature can have a profoundly positive impact on our mental health and overall well-being.

Nature offers a tranquil and rejuvenating environment that can help alleviate stress, reduce anxiety, and promote a sense of inner peace.

Benefits of Time in Nature:

- Stress and Anxiety Reduction: Studies show that exposure to nature can reduce cortisol levels, the stress hormone, and promote a sense of calm and relaxation.

- Mood Improvement: Spending time outdoors can elevate mood and promote feelings of happiness and well-being. The natural beauty of the outdoor environment can inspire feelings of awe and gratitude.

- Increased Creativity and Mental Clarity: Nature has the power to stimulate creativity and promote greater mental clarity. The tranquil and stimulating environment of nature can help shift the mind away from everyday worries and open space for new ideas and perspectives.

How to Enjoy Time in Nature:

1. Go for Outdoor Walks: Explore natural trails in local parks or conservation areas. Walking outdoors allows you to disconnect from the digital world and reconnect with the natural beauty around you.

2. Engage in Outdoor Activities: Try activities such as cycling, kayaking, rock climbing, or bird watching for a more immersive experience in nature.

3. Enjoy Moments of Stillness: Set aside time to simply sit and contemplate nature. Find a quiet spot, such as a bench by a lake or under the shade of a tree, and allow yourself to relax and absorb the serenity of the surroundings.

4. Connect with the Natural Environment: Take a moment to observe the details around you, such as the colors of the leaves, the sounds of the birds, or the feel of the wind on your face. Allow yourself to feel like an integral part of the natural environment.

5. Practice Gratitude: While spending time in nature, take a moment to reflect on the things you are grateful for. Appreciating the beauty and abundance of nature can help cultivate a sense of gratitude and contentment.

By incorporating time in nature into your regular routine, you can reap a host of benefits for mental and emotional health. Take the opportunity to disconnect from the stress of everyday life and reconnect with the beauty and serenity of the natural world around you.

TIP 36: MINDFULNESS PRACTICE

Cultivate mindfulness in your daily activities by paying attention to the present moment with curiosity and acceptance. The practice of mindfulness, or mindfulness, is a powerful tool for cultivating greater awareness and presence in the present moment.

By paying attention to the present moment with curiosity and acceptance, we can reduce stress, increase mental clarity, and promote a sense of inner peace.

Benefits of Mindfulness Practice:

- Stress and Anxiety Reduction: Mindfulness can help reduce levels of stress and anxiety, providing a greater sense of calm and emotional balance.

- Improvement of Concentration: By training the mind to focus on the present moment, mindfulness practice can increase the ability to concentrate and focus.

- Promotion of Emotional Well-Being: Mindfulness can help develop greater emotional resilience, allowing us to deal with life's challenges with more calmness and compassion.

How to Practice Mindfulness:

1. Mindfulness Meditation: Set aside a few minutes every day to practice mindfulness meditation. Sit comfortably, close your eyes, and direct your attention to your breath or the physical sensations of the body.

2. Mindfulness in Daily Activities: Practice mindfulness while engaging in daily activities such as eating, walking, or taking a shower. Pay mindful attention to the sensory details of the experience, such as the taste of food or the feel of water on the skin.

3. Body Scan: Do a mental scan of the body, paying attention to physical sensations and areas of tension. Allow yourself to relax and release any tension that may be present.

4. Mindfulness in Moments of Stress: When feeling stressed or overwhelmed, practice mindfulness by directing your attention to your breath and observing thoughts and emotions without judgment.

5. Gratitude and Appreciation: Cultivate an attitude of gratitude and appreciation for the present moment and the little things in life. Give thanks for positive experiences and acknowledge the beauty around you.

The practice of mindfulness does not require special equipment or advanced skills. Simply dedicate some time and attention to the present moment to reap the lasting benefits of this powerful practice. By cultivating greater awareness and presence in the present moment, you can transform your daily experience into a journey of discovery and personal growth.

TIP 37: MEDIA CONSUMPTION REDUCTION

Limit the time spent on electronic devices and social media, especially before bedtime, to reduce information overload and promote relaxation. Limiting the time spent on electronic devices and social media can be crucial for promoting relaxation and reducing information overload in our daily lives.

Constant exposure to digital media can increase stress, interfere with sleep, and negatively impact our mental health and emotional well-being. Here are some strategies for reducing media consumption and cultivating a greater sense of tranquility:

Benefits of Media Consumption Reduction:

- Improved Sleep Quality: Exposure to blue light emitted by electronic devices can interfere with the natural sleep cycle, making it harder to fall asleep and impairing sleep quality. Limiting screen time before bed can help promote more restful and restorative sleep.

- Stress and Anxiety Reduction: The constant bombardment of information on social media and digital media can lead to a sense of mental and emotional overload. By reducing media consumption, we can decrease stress and anxiety, providing more space for calmness and tranquility.

- Focus on Present Reality: By reducing reliance on electronic devices and social media, we can more fully connect with the world around us and the people in our lives. This allows us to live more in the present moment and enjoy meaningful and authentic experiences.

Strategies for Reducing Media Consumption:

1. Set Time Limits: Set clear limits for the time spent on electronic devices and social media, especially before bedtime. Determine a specific time to disconnect and reserve that time for relaxing and restorative activities.

2. Practice Digital Detachment: Try regular periods of "digital detox," during which you completely disconnect from electronic devices and social media. Use this time to reconnect with offline activities that bring joy and relaxation.

3. Prioritize Face-to-Face Interactions: Instead of communicating exclusively through text messages or social media, seek opportunities to interact in person with friends and family. Prioritize meaningful and authentic relationships outside the digital world.

4. Make Space for Analog Activities: Dedicate time to analog activities, such as reading a physical book, writing in a journal, or practicing a creative hobby. These activities provide a

welcome break from constant digital stimulation and promote a greater connection with oneself.

By consciously reducing digital media consumption in our daily lives, we can create space for calmness, reflection, and meaningful connection with the world around us. By prioritizing balance between the digital world and the real world, we can cultivate a greater sense of tranquility and well-being in our lives.

TIP 38: MASSAGE THERAPY

Schedule regular massage sessions to relax tense muscles and relieve accumulated stress. Scheduling regular massage sessions can be an excellent strategy for relaxing tense muscles and relieving accumulated stress in our body and mind. Massage therapy offers a variety of physical and mental benefits, promoting an overall sense of relaxation and well-being. Here are some of the benefits of massage therapy and how it can help cultivate inner peace:

Benefits of Massage Therapy:

- Stress and Muscle Tension Relief: Massage techniques help release muscle tension and reduce accumulated stress in the body. By relieving muscle tension, we can experience a deep sense of relaxation and tranquility.

- Improved Blood Circulation: Massage increases blood flow to muscles and tissues, promoting the delivery of oxygen and essential nutrients. This can help improve blood circulation and overall body health.

- Pain and Stiffness Reduction: Massage can help alleviate

muscle and joint pain, reducing stiffness and improving range of motion. This can be especially beneficial for people suffering from conditions such as back pain, arthritis, or muscle injuries.

- Promotion of Mental Relaxation: In addition to physical benefits, massage can also promote a state of mental and emotional relaxation. Therapeutic touch and breathing techniques can help calm the mind, reduce anxiety, and promote an overall sense of well-being.

Incorporating Massage Therapy into Your Routine:

- Schedule Regular Sessions: Set aside time regularly for massage sessions, whether weekly, monthly, or as needed, to maintain long-term benefits.

- Communicate Your Needs: Communicate with your massage therapist about your areas of tension and specific concerns, so they can tailor the treatment to your individual needs.

- Combine with Other Relaxation Practices: Complement massage therapy with other relaxation practices, such as meditation, deep breathing, or stretching, to maximize benefits for the body and mind.

- Enjoy Lasting Benefits: The benefits of massage therapy are not limited to the session itself. They can extend beyond the massage table, providing a lasting sense of relaxation and well-being in your everyday life.

By integrating massage therapy into your self-care routine, you can experience a range of benefits for physical and mental health, helping to cultivate a greater sense of inner peace and balance in your life.

TIP 39: THERAPEUTIC WRITING

Keep a journal where you can express your thoughts, feelings, and concerns. Writing can be an effective way to process emotions and find mental clarity. Maintaining a diary where you can express your thoughts, feelings, and concerns can be an effective way to practice therapeutic writing.

Writing offers a powerful way to process emotions, organize thoughts, and find mental clarity. Here are some benefits of therapeutic writing and how it can help cultivate inner peace:

Benefits of Therapeutic Writing:

- Emotional Expression: Writing in a diary allows you to freely express your emotions without judgment or restriction. This can be especially helpful for dealing with intense or complex emotions and finding a healthy outlet to express what you're feeling.

- Self-awareness: Regular practice of therapeutic writing can help you get to know yourself better, identify thought and behavior patterns, and gain insights into yourself and your life experiences.

- Mental Clarity: Writing about your thoughts and concerns can help clear the mind, reduce mental rumination, and promote a sense of calm and tranquility. By putting your thoughts on paper, you can gain a new perspective on issues that concern you.

- Problem Solving: Writing can be an effective tool for problem solving and decision making. By writing about a specific problem or challenge, you can explore different solutions, weigh pros and cons, and come to a more informed conclusion.

Incorporating Therapeutic Writing into Your Routine:

- Establish a Regular Schedule: Set aside regular time to write in your diary, whether it's in the morning to set intentions for the day, in the evening to reflect on your experiences, or whenever you feel the need to process emotions.

- Write Freely: Write without censorship or concern for grammar or cohesion. Let your words flow freely, allowing your thoughts and feelings to be expressed authentically and genuinely.

- Be Consistent: The practice of therapeutic writing is most effective when it is consistent and regular. Make a commitment to write in your diary every day or on specific days of the week to reap the long-term benefits.

- Use as a Self-care Tool: Approach therapeutic writing as a form of self-care and self-exploration. Use your diary as a safe space to process emotions, reflect on experiences, and nurture your mental and emotional health.

By incorporating therapeutic writing into your daily routine, you can enjoy a variety of benefits for mental and emotional health, helping to cultivate a greater sense of inner peace, mental clarity, and overall well-being in your life.

TIP 40: YOGA PRACTICE

Attend yoga classes or practice at home to strengthen the body, increase flexibility, and calm the mind. Attending yoga classes or practicing at home can be an excellent strategy to strengthen the body, increase flexibility, and calm the mind.

Yoga is an ancient practice that combines physical postures, breathing techniques, and meditation to promote balance and well-being in all aspects of life. Here are some benefits of yoga practice and how it can help cultivate inner peace:

Benefits of Yoga Practice:

- Muscle Strengthening: Yoga postures are designed to strengthen the muscles of the body, including arms, legs, abdomen, and back. Yoga helps tone and define the body holistically, promoting an overall sense of strength and vitality.

- Increased Flexibility: Yoga emphasizes stretching and flexibility, helping to improve range of motion and prevent injuries. As you practice regularly, you'll notice that your flexibility gradually increases, allowing you to move more easily and freely in your daily life.

- Mental Health Promotion: The combination of breathing techniques, meditation, and movement in yoga can help calm the mind, reduce stress, and promote a sense of inner calm. Regular yoga practice can help you cultivate greater awareness of the present moment and find peace amidst the chaos of everyday life.

- Improved Emotional Balance: Yoga teaches the art of balancing body, mind, and spirit, helping to cultivate a state of emotional balance and well-being. By practicing yoga regularly, you can develop skills to cope with stress, anxiety, and other challenging emotions more effectively.

Incorporating Yoga Practice into Your Routine:

- Find a Style that Works for You: There are many different styles of yoga, from gentle and relaxing to dynamic and challenging. Try out different styles to find what resonates best with you and your individual needs.

- Establish a Regular Routine: Set aside regular time to practice yoga, whether it's a few times a week in formal classes or daily in your own home practice. Consistency is key to reaping the long-term benefits of yoga.

- Adjust Your Practice to Your Needs: Don't be afraid to adapt your yoga practice according to your needs and physical limitations. Listen to your body and make adjustments as necessary to ensure a safe and rewarding practice.

- Enjoy the Benefits Beyond the Mat: The benefits of yoga are not limited to your practice on the mat. Bring the teachings of yoga into your everyday life, cultivating an attitude of compassion, gratitude, and acceptance in all areas of your life.

By incorporating yoga practice into your daily routine, you can enjoy a variety of benefits for the body, mind, and spirit, helping to cultivate a greater sense of inner peace, emotional balance, and overall well-being in your life.

TIP 41: HEALTHY EATING

Prioritize a balanced diet, rich in fruits, vegetables, whole grains, and lean proteins. Healthy eating can provide the necessary nutrients to sustain both body and mind. Prioritizing a balanced diet, rich in fruits, vegetables, whole grains, and lean proteins is crucial for nourishing both body and mind.

Healthy eating provides the necessary nutrients to sustain energy, promote well-being, and cultivate inner peace. Here are some benefits of healthy eating and how it can contribute to your overall balance:

Benefits of Healthy Eating:

- Provision of Essential Nutrients: A balanced diet provides a variety of essential nutrients, including vitamins, minerals, proteins, and fibers, which are needed to maintain health and proper body function.

- Support for Mental Health: The connection between diet and mental health is powerful. Nutrient-rich foods, such as omega-3 fatty acids, B vitamins, and antioxidants, can help promote mental health, reduce stress, and improve mood.

- Weight Management: Healthy eating, combined with regular physical activity, can help maintain a healthy body weight and prevent excessive weight gain. Maintaining a healthy weight is important for both physical and emotional health.

- Strengthening the Immune System: Nutrient-rich foods, such as fruits, vegetables, and lean proteins, contain antioxidants and other compounds that help strengthen the immune system, reducing the risk of diseases and infections.

- Increased Energy and Vitality: Healthy eating provides the energy needed to sustain daily activities, promoting a sense of vitality and well-being throughout the day.

Incorporating Healthy Eating into Your Routine:

- Diversify Your Diet: Consume a variety of foods from all food groups, including fruits, vegetables, whole grains, lean proteins, and healthy fats. The more colorful and diverse your plate, the more nutrients you'll be consuming.

- Stay Hydrated: Drink plenty of water throughout the day to keep the body hydrated and support proper bodily functions. Avoid sugary drinks and opt for water, herbal teas, or fruit-infused water instead.

- Plan Your Meals: Take time to plan your meals and snacks in advance, ensuring that you have healthy options readily available. This can help avoid impulsive food choices and maintain a balanced diet.

- Avoid Processed Foods: Limit the intake of processed foods, such as those high in added sugars, trans fats, and artificial additives. Opt for natural and minimally processed foods whenever possible.

- Practice Moderation: Enjoy your favorite foods occasionally, but in controlled portions. Allowing yourself moderate indulgences can help maintain balance and satisfaction in your eating habits.

By prioritizing healthy eating in your daily life, you can reap a variety of benefits for physical, mental, and emotional health, helping to cultivate a greater sense of inner peace, vitality, and overall well-being in your life.

TIP 42: ESTABLISH BOUNDARIES

Learning to say no when necessary and establishing healthy boundaries in your relationships and commitments is essential for protecting your energy and well-being. Here are some reasons why establishing boundaries is important and how it can contribute to your inner peace:

Importance of Establishing Boundaries:

- Energy Protection: Setting clear boundaries allows you to protect your energy and reserve time and space to take care of yourself. This helps avoid overload and burnout, allowing you to feel more balanced and centered.

- Promotion of Self-Respect: By establishing healthy boundaries, you are affirming your own worth and respecting your needs and desires. This strengthens your self-esteem and self-confidence, allowing you to feel more secure in your interactions with others.

- Improvement of Relationships: Setting clear boundaries in your relationships can help improve communication and foster healthier, more satisfying relationships. This can prevent conflicts and resentments, allowing you to build more authentic and meaningful connections with others.

- Stress Reduction: By setting appropriate boundaries, you can reduce the stress and anxiety associated with feeling overwhelmed or overextended. This allows you to focus on your priorities and take care of yourself more effectively.

How to Establish Boundaries:

- Identify Your Needs: First, recognize your own needs, desires, and limitations. This can help you determine which boundaries are necessary to protect your health and well-being.

- Communicate Clearly and Respectfully: Communicate your boundaries clearly, directly, and respectfully with others. Be assertive in expressing your needs and don't be afraid to say no when necessary.

- Set Consequences: Establish clear consequences for disrespecting your boundaries and be prepared to enforce them if necessary. This can help reinforce your boundaries and ensure they are respected by others.

- Be Consistent: Stay firm in your boundaries and be consistent in their enforcement. This may require practice and patience, but over time, you will feel more confident and comfortable in establishing and maintaining healthy boundaries.

By establishing healthy boundaries in your life, you can protect your energy, promote self-respect, and improve your relationships, helping you cultivate a greater sense of inner peace and balance in all areas of your life.

TIP 43: PROGRESSIVE MUSCLE RELAXATION PRACTICE:

Try progressive muscle relaxation techniques, where you sequentially tense and relax the muscles of the body to relieve accumulated tension. This technique can be an effective strategy for relieving accumulated tension and promoting a sense of calm and relaxation. Here's how you can practice this technique and the benefits it can offer:

How to Practice Progressive Muscle Relaxation:

1. Find a Quiet Environment: Choose a calm and quiet location where you can sit or lie down comfortably without interruptions.

2. Relax Your Breathing: Begin by breathing deeply and slowly, allowing your breath to become natural and rhythmic.

3. Focus on the Muscles: Start the progressive tension of the muscles, beginning from the feet and gradually moving up to the head. For each muscle group, deliberately tense them for a few seconds and then completely relax them.

4. Maintain Body Awareness: As you focus on each muscle group, be present and aware of the physical sensations that arise. Notice the difference between tension and relaxation in each part of the body.

5. Progress Gradually: Continue working through the body, from the feet to the head, tensing and relaxing the muscles as needed. Pay special attention to areas where you tend to accumulate more tension, such as the shoulders, neck, and jaw.

6. Stay Relaxed: After completing the sequence of progressive muscle relaxation, allow yourself to remain in a state of relaxation for a few moments, enjoying the sense of calm and tranquility you have created.

Benefits of Progressive Muscle Relaxation:

- Muscle Tension Relief: By tensing and relaxing the muscles of the body, you can release accumulated tension and reduce muscle stiffness, promoting a deep sense of relaxation.

- Stress and Anxiety Reduction: Practicing progressive muscle relaxation can help calm the mind and reduce symptoms associated with stress and anxiety, such as rapid heart rate and shallow breathing.

- Improvement in Sleep Quality: By relaxing the body and calming the mind, progressive muscle relaxation can help improve sleep quality, facilitating falling asleep and promoting deeper and more restorative sleep.

- Promotion of General Well-being: Incorporating progressive muscle relaxation into your daily routine can help promote a greater sense of overall well-being, increasing your ability to cope with stress and the demands of daily life.

Try to reserve a few minutes every day to practice progressive muscle relaxation and observe the benefits this technique can bring to your physical, mental, and emotional health.

TIP 44: CREATIVE VISUALIZATION

Dedicate a few minutes each day to visualize a calm and relaxing place or situation. Creative visualization can help reduce stress and promote feelings of calm and inner peace. Dedicating a few minutes each day to practice creative visualization can be a powerful technique for reducing stress and promoting feelings of calm and inner peace. Here's how you can practice creative visualization and the benefits it can offer:

How to Practice Creative Visualization:

1. Find a Quiet Environment: Choose a calm and quiet location where you can sit or lie down comfortably, without interruptions.

2. Relax the Body and Mind: Begin by breathing deeply and relaxing the muscles of the body, allowing your mind to calm and quiet.

3. Choose a Relaxing Scene: Close your eyes and begin to visualize a place or situation that brings feelings of peace and tranquility. This could be a sunny beach, a serene forest, or even a quiet garden.

4. Explore the Details: As you imagine your relaxing scene, focus on all the sensory details. Imagine the gentle sounds of the environment, the pleasant scents in the air, and the comforting sensations in your body.

5. Engage in the Experience: Allow yourself to fully immerse in the experience of the visualization, soaking in the calm and serenity it evokes. Let yourself feel present and engaged in the scene, as if you were truly there.

6. Stay for a While: Stay in the visualization for as long as you wish, allowing the feelings of peace and tranquility to strengthen within you. When you're ready, open your eyes and return to the present, carrying with you the feelings of calm you've cultivated.

Benefits of Creative Visualization:

- Stress and Anxiety Reduction: Creative visualization can help calm the mind and reduce symptoms associated with stress and anxiety, offering a relaxing break from the daily hustle and bustle.

- Promotion of Deep Relaxation: By immersing yourself in a relaxing scene, you allow your body and mind to enter a state of deep relaxation, promoting a sense of calm and well-being.

- Strengthening of Mental Resilience: Regular practice of creative visualization can help strengthen your mental resilience, providing you with a powerful tool to cope with life's challenges and adversities.

- Cultivation of Inner Peace: By cultivating a sense of inner peace through creative visualization, you can enhance your quality of life and enjoy greater harmony and balance in all areas of your life.

Try to reserve a few minutes every day to practice creative visualization and discover the transformative benefits it can bring to your overall health and well-being.

TIP 45: ESTABLISH A SLEEP ROUTINE

Prioritize a consistent sleep routine, with regular bed and wake times. Adequate sleep is crucial for both physical and mental health. Prioritizing a consistent sleep routine is essential for promoting physical and mental health. Here are some tips for establishing a healthy sleep routine:

Tips for a Healthy Sleep Routine:

1. Regular Schedule: Try to go to bed and wake up at the same times every day, including weekends. This helps regulate your body's biological clock and promotes more consistent sleep.

2. Create a Comfortable Environment: Ensure that your bedroom is conducive to sleep, with a comfortable temperature, minimal light, and a mattress and pillows suited to your comfort.

3. Avoid Stimulants Before Bed: Avoid stimulants such as caffeine and nicotine before bedtime, and limit the use of electronic devices, such as smartphones and computers, at least an hour before bedtime.

4. Practice Relaxation: Dedicate some time before bed to relax

and unwind. This can include taking a warm bath, practicing breathing techniques or meditation, or simply reading a relaxing book.

5. Avoid Heavy Meals: Avoid heavy meals and heavy snacks before bedtime, as this can cause digestive discomfort and make it difficult to sleep.

6. Exercise Regularly: Engage in regular exercise, but avoid intense activities close to bedtime. Regular exercise can help promote deeper and more restorative sleep.

7. Limit Naps: If you feel the need to take a nap during the day, limit it to 20-30 minutes and avoid taking it too late, as this can affect your ability to sleep at night.

8. Stay Comfortable: Make sure your mattress and pillows provide the necessary support and comfort for a good night's sleep. Replace them regularly, if necessary.

Benefits of a Healthy Sleep Routine:

- Improved Cognitive Performance: Adequate sleep is essential for cognitive function, including concentration, memory, and decision-making.

- Mood Enhancement: A good night's sleep is associated with better mood and greater ability to cope with stress and negative emotions.

- Physical Health: Adequate sleep plays a crucial role in physical health, including immune function, metabolism, and hormonal regulation.

- Muscle Recovery: During sleep, the body has the opportunity to recover and repair muscle tissues, promoting more effective recovery after physical exercise.

Prioritizing a healthy sleep routine can have a significant impact on your overall health and well-being. Try implementing these tips into your daily routine and observe the transformative benefits that adequate sleep can bring to your life.

TIP 46: ENGAGE IN HOBBIES

Set aside time for activities that bring you joy and satisfaction, such as creative hobbies, sports, or music. Engaging in enjoyable activities can relieve stress and promote happiness. Setting aside time for activities that bring you joy and satisfaction is essential for your emotional and mental well-being. Here are some ways to engage in hobbies and reap the positive benefits:

Benefits of Engaging in Hobbies:

1. Stress Relief: Participating in activities you love can be an excellent way to relieve accumulated stress and tension throughout the day.

2. Escape from Routine: Hobbies offer a welcome break from the daily routine, allowing you to disconnect from work and everyday life concerns.

3. Creative Expression: Creative hobbies, such as painting, writing, or music, offer an outlet for creative expression, allowing you to express yourself in unique and meaningful ways.

4. Self-Discovery: Exploring new hobbies can help you discover new passions and interests, as well as learn more about yourself and your abilities.

5. Mood Improvement: Engaging in activities you love can increase your levels of happiness and improve your overall mood.

Tips for Finding and Enjoying Hobbies:

- Try New Things: Be open to trying different hobbies and activities until you find ones that truly resonate with you.

- Make Time: Regularly schedule time in your agenda to dedicate to your hobbies, even if it's just for a few minutes each day.

- Share with Others: Find communities or groups of people who share your interests and hobbies, so you can connect and learn from others.

- Don't Pressure Yourself: Remember that the goal of hobbies is to enjoy and have fun, so don't worry about performance or perfect results.

- Variety is Key: Try a variety of different hobbies to keep things interesting and avoid boredom.

- Balance: Find a healthy balance between your hobbies and other areas of your life, so you can fully enjoy all your activities.

No matter what your interests or passions are, setting aside time to engage in hobbies is an important part of taking care of yourself and promoting your overall well-being. Allow yourself to explore, experiment, and enjoy activities that make you happy and fulfilled.

TIP 47: AROMATHERAPY PRACTICE

Experience relaxing essential oils such as lavender, chamomile, or bergamot to promote calmness and relaxation. Experimenting with relaxing essential oils is an effective way to promote calmness and relaxation in your daily life. Here's how aromatherapy can benefit your health and well-being:

Benefits of Aromatherapy:

1. Stress Relief: Certain essential oils, such as lavender, chamomile, and bergamot, have relaxing properties that can help alleviate stress and anxiety.

2. Mood Enhancement: Pleasant aromas can have a positive impact on your mood, uplifting spirits, and reducing feelings of sadness or irritability.

3. Sleep Promotion: Some essential oils, like lavender, are known for their sedative properties, which can help promote deeper and more restorative sleep.

4. Pain and Tension Relief: Certain essential oils have analgesic and anti-inflammatory properties that can help alleviate muscle

pain and tension.

5. Improved Concentration: Some scents, like peppermint or rosemary, are known to increase mental clarity and concentration, being useful during work or study.

How to Practice Aromatherapy:

- Oil Diffusers: Use an essential oil diffuser to disperse aromas into the air, creating a relaxing atmosphere in your home or office.

- Massage: Add a few drops of essential oil to a carrier oil, such as coconut oil or jojoba oil, and use it to massage the body, relieving pain and tension.

- Relaxing Bath: Add a few drops of essential oil to bathwater to create a relaxing and invigorating bath experience.

- Direct Inhalation: Place a few drops of essential oil on a tissue or aromatherapy pillow and breathe deeply to enjoy therapeutic benefits.

- Room Sprays: Create your own room spray with water and essential oils to refresh and purify the air around you.

Experiment with different essential oils and application methods to discover what works best for you and how to incorporate aromatherapy into your daily routine to promote relaxation, well-being, and emotional balance.

TIP 48: SOCIAL CONNECTION

Cultivate meaningful relationships with friends and family. Social support can be an important source of comfort and support during stressful times. Cultivating meaningful relationships with friends and family is crucial for your emotional and mental well-being. Here's how social connection can benefit your health:

Benefits of Social Connection:

1. Emotional Support: Having friends and family whom you can share your joys and concerns with can provide valuable emotional support during difficult times.

2. Stress Reduction: Simply spending time with loved ones can help reduce stress and anxiety levels, providing comfort and support.

3. Increased Happiness: Positive and rewarding relationships are associated with higher levels of happiness and life satisfaction.

4. Improved Mental Health: Social connection is linked to a lower incidence of depression, anxiety, and other mental health issues.

5. Strengthened Immune System: Healthy relationships can strengthen the immune system, making it more resistant to illness and infections.

How to Cultivate Meaningful Relationships:

- Prioritize Time Together: Make a conscious effort to spend quality time with your loved ones, even if it's just for a quick phone call or a shared meal.

- Be Present: Be there for your friends and family when they need support, listen attentively, and offer your support in a caring and compassionate manner.

- Share Experiences: Seek opportunities to create memories and share meaningful experiences together, whether through travel, shared hobbies, or simply spending quality time together.

- Express Gratitude: Demonstrate appreciation and gratitude for the relationships in your life, acknowledging and valuing the important role your loved ones play in your well-being.

- Be Authentic: Cultivate relationships based on authenticity, honesty, and mutual trust, where you can be yourself without judgment.

- Engage in Communities: Get involved in groups or communities with similar interests, which can be a great way to meet new people and build new meaningful relationships.

Remember that social connection is a vital part of a healthy and happy life. Prioritize your relationships and invest time and energy in cultivating meaningful connections with those who are important to you.

TIP 49: LEARN TO DELEGATE

Don't be afraid to delegate tasks when necessary and ask for help when needed. Overloading yourself with responsibilities can contribute to stress, so learn to share the burden when possible. Learning to delegate tasks is an essential skill for managing stress and maintaining a healthy balance between work, personal life, and well-being. Here are some reasons why delegation is important and how you can implement it in your life:

Importance of Delegation:

1. Reduction of Overload: Trying to do everything alone can lead to overload and burnout. Delegating tasks allows for more equitable distribution of work and alleviates the burden on your shoulders.

2. Increased Efficiency: By delegating tasks to people with specific skills, you can make the most of individual talents and complete tasks more efficiently and effectively.

3. Focus on Priorities: Delegating less important tasks or those outside your area of expertise allows you to focus on tasks that

are more critical and strategic to your goals.

4. Skill Development: Delegating tasks can be an opportunity for personal and professional growth and development, both for yourself and for the people you delegate to.

How to Delegate Effectively:

1. Identify Suitable Tasks for Delegation: Evaluate your responsibilities and identify tasks that can be easily transferred to others, considering their skills and areas of expertise.

2. Choose the Right People: When delegating tasks, select the most suitable people for the job, considering their skills, experience, and availability.

3. Communicate Clear Expectations: Ensure clear communication of expectations regarding the delegated task, including deadlines, quality standards, and any specific guidance needed.

4. Provide Support and Resources: Ensure that the people you delegate to have the necessary resources and support to successfully complete the task. Be available to answer questions and offer guidance as needed.

5. Delegate Appropriate Authority: When delegating tasks, ensure that you delegate not only responsibilities but also the authority needed to make decisions related to the task.

6. Monitor Progress: Stay involved in the process by monitoring the progress of the task and providing feedback and support as needed.

Learning to delegate effectively can be a transformative skill that can help you achieve your goals more efficiently and reduce stress in your daily life. Don't be afraid to ask for help and share the burden when necessary—you may be surprised by how much you can accomplish when working as a team.

TIP 50: PRACTICE SELF-CARE

Regularly set aside time to take care of yourself, whether through relaxing baths, reading, or any other activity that brings you pleasure and relaxation.

Self-Care Practice:

Self-care practice is essential for maintaining emotional, physical, and mental balance amidst the demands of daily life. Set aside time regularly to take care of yourself and recharge your energy. Here are some ways to incorporate self-care into your routine:

1. Prioritize Time for Yourself: Set aside time regularly to engage in activities that bring you pleasure and relaxation. This may include taking relaxing baths, reading a book, practicing hobbies, or simply resting and recharging.

2. Listen to Your Body and Mind's Needs: Pay attention to the signals your body and mind are sending and respond to them with kindness and compassion. Take regular breaks throughout the day to stretch, breathe deeply, and relax.

3. Take Care of Your Physical Health: In addition to caring for your mental and emotional health, don't forget about your physical health. Maintain a balanced diet, exercise regularly, and ensure you get enough sleep every night.

4. Establish Healthy Boundaries: Learn to say no when necessary and establish healthy boundaries in your relationships and commitments. Respecting your own limits is essential to protect your energy and well-being.

5. Cultivate Moments of Calm: Find moments throughout the day to cultivate calm and relaxation. This may include practices such as meditation, mindful breathing, or simply taking short breaks to slow down and reconnect with yourself.

6. Be Gentle with Yourself: Practice self-compassion and be gentle with yourself, especially in moments of difficulty. Recognize that you are human and allow yourself to fail, learn, and grow from your experiences.

7. Seek Support When Needed: Don't be afraid to ask for help and support when you need it. Talking to friends, family, or a mental health professional can provide the necessary support to face challenges and take care of yourself.

Remember that self-care is not a luxury but an essential need for your overall well-being. Prioritize yourself and set aside time to take care of yourself, as this not only benefits you but also those around you.

TIP 51: PRACTICE ACCEPTANCE

Learn to accept the things you cannot change and focus your energy on those within your control. Acceptance can bring inner peace by releasing resistance to reality.

This practice of acceptance is a powerful journey towards inner peace and emotional balance. Recognizing reality as it is, without trying to change it or resist it, allows us to find serenity even in the most challenging circumstances.

By cultivating acceptance, we also learn to practice non-judgment, both towards ourselves and others, enabling us to live with more compassion and understanding.

Releasing the need for control helps us trust in the flow of life and opens us up to new possibilities, while finding meaning in adversity, turning challenges into opportunities for growth and learning.

Gratitude becomes a fundamental practice, allowing us to focus on the blessings present in our lives, even when facing difficulties.

Being present in the moment helps us find calm and inner peace, regardless of concerns about the past or the future.

Through these practices, we can cultivate a life of serenity, resilience, and contentment, finding inner peace even amidst the storms of life.

TIP 52: TAKE BREAKS DURING THE DAY

Integrate small relaxation breaks throughout the day where you can disconnect, take deep breaths, and recharge your energy.

Integrating small breaks during the day is an effective way to reduce stress and cultivate inner peace. Taking a few moments to disconnect from the demands of daily life, take deep breaths, and recharge your energy can make a big difference in your emotional and mental well-being.

During these breaks, you can choose to simply close your eyes and take deep breaths, practice some mindful breathing exercises, or even take a quick walk outdoors to change your environment and clear your mind.

These breaks don't need to be long or elaborate; the important thing is that they provide a moment of calm and renewal amidst the hustle and bustle of the day. By incorporating these breaks into your daily routine, you can help reduce accumulated stress and promote an overall sense of well-being and balance.

TIP 53: STIMULATE CREATIVITY

Explore your creativity through activities such as painting, writing, music, or crafts. Creative expression can be a powerful way to relieve stress and promote emotional well-being.

Stimulating creativity is an excellent way to nourish your soul and promote inner peace. By engaging in creative activities such as painting, writing, music, or crafts, you can unleash your imagination, express yourself freely, and find a healthy outlet for the stress and worries of daily life.

Creative expression provides a safe space to explore your emotions, thoughts, and experiences in a unique and personal way. Painting on a blank canvas, writing in a journal, or composing a piece of music can be powerful ways to process complex emotions, find mental clarity, and promote a sense of emotional well-being.

Additionally, creativity can help stimulate the mind, boost self-esteem, and provide a sense of personal accomplishment. By allowing yourself to explore your creativity, you may discover new passions, hidden talents, and a greater connection with yourself and the world around you.

Therefore, set aside time regularly to engage in creative activities that inspire you and bring joy. Don't worry about the end result; the creative process itself is what matters. Allow yourself to experiment, make mistakes, and grow as you dive into the wonderful world of creativity.

TIP 54: DEVELOP RESILIENCE

Cultivate a mindset of resilience, seeing challenges as opportunities for growth and learning. Resilience helps us face life's challenges with courage and determination.

Developing resilience is crucial for effectively and constructively dealing with life's challenges. Instead of being overwhelmed by difficulties and setbacks, resilience empowers us to confront challenges with courage, determination, and mental flexibility.

A resilient mindset allows us to view challenges as opportunities for growth and learning. Rather than getting stuck in failure or adversity, we seek to extract valuable lessons from each experience, strengthening ourselves in the process. Resilience teaches us to adapt to ever-changing circumstances and find creative solutions to the problems we face.

To develop resilience, it's important to cultivate a range of skills and positive attitudes:

1. Acceptance of Reality: Recognizing and accepting the reality of the situation, even when it's challenging, is the first step in building resilience. This allows us to deal with the situation

objectively and seek effective solutions.

2. Focus on Control: Concentrating on things we can control and letting go of those beyond our control is essential for developing resilience. This helps us direct our energy to areas where we can make a difference and avoid wasting it on unproductive worries.

3. Adaptation and Flexibility: Resilience involves being able to adapt to life's changes and challenges. This requires mental flexibility and the ability to adjust our strategies as needed to deal with new circumstances.

4. Self-Confidence: Having confidence in our abilities and capabilities strengthens us in the face of adversity. Cultivating a positive self-image and believing in our ability to overcome challenges is essential for developing resilience.

5. Support Network: Relying on the support of friends, family, and other community members is crucial for building resilience. Having people we trust and can turn to in difficult times helps us face challenges with more confidence and determination.

By developing these skills and attitudes, we can strengthen our resilience and become better equipped to handle life's ups and downs. Rather than being knocked down by challenges, we can rise up stronger and more resilient, ready to face whatever the future holds.

TIP 55: PRACTICE COMPASSION

Be kind to yourself and others. Practicing compassion can promote feelings of connection and empathy, reducing stress and promoting inner peace.

Practicing compassion is essential for promoting inner peace and cultivating healthy relationships with yourself and others. Compassion involves being kind, loving, and compassionate, both to yourself and to others, especially in times of difficulty and suffering.

When we practice compassion, we recognize and accept our own imperfections and weaknesses, treating ourselves with kindness and understanding instead of criticism and self-criticism. This allows us to cultivate a more positive and compassionate relationship with ourselves, thereby promoting inner peace and self-acceptance.

Additionally, practicing compassion towards others helps us develop empathy and human connection, fostering deeper and more meaningful relationships. By recognizing and responding to others' needs with kindness and compassion, we strengthen bonds of empathy and solidarity, creating an environment of mutual support and understanding.

Compassion also plays an important role in reducing stress and emotional suffering. By cultivating an attitude of compassion towards ourselves and others, we can alleviate the burden of self-criticism, guilt, and judgment, thus promoting greater emotional and mental well-being.

To practice compassion in your daily life, you can:

- Cultivate self-compassion, treating yourself with kindness and understanding in times of difficulty and suffering.

- Develop empathy and understanding towards others, recognizing and responding to their needs with kindness and compassion.

- Practice acts of kindness and generosity, both to yourself and to others, thereby promoting an environment of mutual support and understanding.

- Cultivate an attitude of acceptance and compassion towards the imperfections and difficulties of life, recognizing that we all face challenges and struggles on our journey.

By practicing compassion in your daily life, you can promote feelings of inner peace, human connection, and emotional well-being, thus creating a more compassionate and supportive world for yourself and others.

TIP 56: SET REALISTIC GOALS

Set achievable and realistic goals for yourself, breaking down big tasks into smaller steps and celebrating your progress along the way.

Setting realistic goals is essential for promoting inner peace and achieving a sense of personal fulfillment. By defining achievable and realistic goals, you create a clear framework for your progress and empower yourself to move towards your dreams consistently and sustainably.

When your goals are realistic, you avoid the burden of unrealistic expectations and excessive pressure on yourself. Instead, you focus on goals that are within your reach and can be achieved with adequate effort and dedication. This reduces the stress and anxiety associated with unattainable goals, allowing you to feel more confident and motivated on your journey.

Additionally, setting realistic goals also helps to break down big tasks into smaller and more manageable steps, facilitating gradual progress towards your objectives. By breaking your goals into smaller, achievable steps, you create a clear and tangible action plan that guides you on your path to success.

When setting realistic goals, it's important to celebrate your progress along the way. Recognize and celebrate your achievements, no matter how small, and use these moments as a source of ongoing inspiration and motivation. This not only strengthens your confidence and self-esteem but also reinforces your commitment to your goals and fuels your desire to achieve even more.

In summary, setting realistic goals is essential for promoting inner peace, reducing stress, and achieving a sense of personal fulfillment. By defining achievable goals and breaking down big tasks into smaller steps, you create a tangible action plan that empowers you to move towards your dreams consistently and sustainably.

TIP 57: PRACTICE ACTIVE LISTENING

When engaging in conversations with others, practice active listening by giving full attention to what is being said without judgment or interruption.

Practicing active listening is an essential skill for promoting inner peace and cultivating healthy, meaningful relationships. When engaging in conversations with others, it's easy to get lost in our own thoughts and concerns, failing to truly listen to what the other person is saying. However, by practicing active listening, we can connect more deeply with others, demonstrate empathy and understanding, and strengthen our interpersonal bonds.

Active listening involves giving full attention to what the other person is saying, without distractions or interruptions. This means making eye contact, using receptive body language, and showing genuine interest in what is being said. By fully focusing on the person who is speaking, you show respect and value their perspective, creating an environment of open and confident communication.

Additionally, active listening also involves demonstrating

empathy and understanding towards the other person's feelings and experiences. This means not only listening to their words but also acknowledging and validating their emotions, showing genuine concern and care. By emotionally connecting with others in this way, you strengthen your relationships and promote a sense of unity and mutual support.

Practicing active listening can also bring significant benefits to your own inner peace. By focusing on the present moment and truly connecting with others, you may experience a sense of calm and inner contentment. Additionally, by demonstrating empathy and compassion towards others, you enhance your own ability to relate to others and cultivate healthy, meaningful relationships.

In summary, practicing active listening is a powerful skill that can promote inner peace, strengthen relationships, and improve overall quality of life. When engaging in conversations with others, make a conscious effort to give full attention, demonstrate empathy and understanding, and create a safe and welcoming space for open and honest communication.

TIP 58: LEARN
TO SAY NO

Recognize your own limits and learn to say no to excessive demands or those that are not aligned with your priorities and values.

Learning to say no is essential for preserving your energy, protecting your boundaries, and cultivating inner peace. Often, we feel social or internal pressure to meet the expectations of others, even if it means overwhelming our own physical, emotional, and mental resources. However, by recognizing your own limits and learning to say no assertively and respectfully, you can promote your own health and well-being.

Saying no does not mean being selfish or insensitive to others. On the contrary, it is a form of self-care and authenticity. By setting clear boundaries and communicating your needs honestly, you build more authentic and healthy relationships based on mutual respect and understanding. Additionally, learning to say no can also help you prioritize your own goals and values, allowing you to focus on what is truly important to you.

However, learning to say no can be challenging, especially if you are accustomed to putting others' needs before your own. Here are some tips to help you learn to say no effectively and respectfully:

1. Know your limits: Take time to reflect on your own needs, values, and priorities. Identify what your personal limits are and what you are willing to accept in terms of external demands.

2. Practice assertiveness: When saying no, be clear, firm, and assertive in your communication. Use direct and objective language to express your refusal, without over-apologizing or making excuses.

3. Offer alternatives: If possible, offer alternatives or suggestions that may help meet the other person's needs in a way that is more compatible with your own limits and priorities.

4. Be consistent: Stick to your boundaries and decisions, even if it means facing resistance or disapproval from others. Remember that you have the right to prioritize your own health and well-being.

5. Practice self-care: Set aside time to take care of yourself and recharge your energy regularly. Prioritize activities that help you relax, rejuvenate, and regain emotional balance.

By learning to say no effectively and respectfully, you strengthen your self-esteem, protect your energy, and promote greater inner peace. Remember that it is perfectly acceptable to establish healthy boundaries and advocate for your own needs and values.

TIP 59: CULTIVATE MOMENTS OF SILENCE

Set aside moments of silence in your daily life to disconnect from external noise and connect with yourself. Silence can be a powerful source of clarity and tranquility.

Cultivating moments of silence amidst the hustle and bustle of everyday life is essential for nurturing our inner peace, promoting reflection, and restoring our emotional balance. In a world filled with constant stimuli, silence offers a quiet refuge where we can reconnect with our own essence and find calm amidst the chaos.

Silence not only provides us with a much-needed respite from the noise of the external world but also allows us to dive deeply into our inner world. It is in these moments of quietude that we can hear the gentle voice of our intuition, reflect on our deepest thoughts and feelings, and find clarity amidst confusion.

Additionally, silence has the power to teach us valuable lessons about the importance of presence and mindfulness. When we allow ourselves to be silent, we learn to be truly present in the moment, without distractions or concerns about the past or the future. This allows us to experience a sense of peace and serenity that cannot be found anywhere else.

To cultivate moments of silence in your daily life, you can start by incorporating practices such as meditation, contemplation, nature walks, or simply sitting in silence for a few minutes every day. Set aside time regularly to disconnect from external noise, turn off your electronic devices, and connect with yourself in a space of calm and tranquility.

Remember that silence is not just the absence of sound but an opportunity to dive deeply into our own essence and find peace within ourselves. By cultivating moments of silence in your daily life, you strengthen your connection with yourself, promote greater mental clarity, and nurture your inner peace.

TIP 60: PRACTICE FORGIVENESS

Release past resentments and grievances by practicing forgiveness, both for others and for yourself. Forgiveness is a way to let go of the emotional baggage of the past and make room for inner peace.

Practicing forgiveness is a powerful act of self-love and emotional liberation. When we carry resentments and grievances from the past, we are perpetually bound to these negative emotions, which can negatively impact our inner peace and emotional well-being. However, by practicing forgiveness, we can break these emotional bonds and find a true sense of freedom and peace.

Forgiveness doesn't necessarily mean forgetting or excusing someone else's harmful behavior. Instead, forgiveness is a conscious choice to release the emotional weight of the past and move forward with compassion and acceptance. This not only benefits the person being forgiven but also brings significant benefits to the one forgiving.

By practicing forgiveness, we are freeing ourselves from the emotional baggage we carry and making room for more positive feelings such as compassion, love, and peace. This allows us to live more fully in the present moment rather than being stuck in the past. Additionally, forgiveness helps us cultivate healthier and more meaningful relationships as it allows us to let go of resentments and foster greater empathy and understanding in our interactions with others.

It's important to note that forgiveness is not an easy process and may take time and practice. It may require significant internal work to acknowledge and release the negative emotions associated with the past. However, the benefits of forgiveness—both for our emotional health and overall well-being—are well worth the effort.

When practicing forgiveness, remember to include yourself in the process. Often, we are harder on ourselves than we are on others, and self-forgiveness is essential for cultivating true inner peace. By releasing resentments and grievances, both towards others and ourselves, we can pave the way for a fuller, more compassionate, and peaceful life.

As we explore strategies for managing stress and cultivating inner peace, we discover a diverse set of tools and practices that can help us navigate life's complexities in a more balanced and harmonious way. From practicing gratitude to forgiveness, each of these techniques offers a unique opportunity to promote greater emotional well-being and a deeper sense of inner tranquility.

It's important to recognize that the path to inner peace is not linear and may require ongoing effort and commitment. However, by incorporating these strategies into our daily lives and cultivating an attitude of openness and acceptance, we can gradually transform our life experience and create an internal space where calm and serenity can flourish.

By practicing self-care, compassion, and gratitude, we not only benefit ourselves but also those around us. We cultivate healthier relationships, promote a more productive work environment, and contribute to a more compassionate and supportive community.

As we continue on the journey toward emotional well-being and inner peace, it's essential to remember that each individual is unique, and what works for one person may not work for another. Therefore, it's crucial to explore and experiment with different techniques, adapting them to our individual needs and preferences.

Additionally, it's important to remember that the process of cultivating inner peace is ongoing and dynamic. Like practicing a musical instrument or honing a skill, it requires time, patience, and dedication to develop a lasting state of serenity.

Throughout this process, it's normal to encounter challenges and setbacks. However, it's important not to become discouraged in the face of difficulties but rather to see each obstacle as an opportunity for growth and learning.

Therefore, I encourage you to continue exploring, experimenting, and committing to practices that promote your emotional well-being and inner peace. Be kind to yourself during this process, and remember that each small step toward self-care and self-compassion is a victory in itself.

May we walk together on this journey, supporting each other and sharing our experiences as we strive for a fuller, more balanced, and meaningful life.

Now that we've come this far, it's essential for you, the reader, to know that none of this will yield results if you don't improve your sleep quality and, consequently, increase your productivity. Everything is related to good sleep quality aligned with physical activity, good nutrition, and the other tips that have been provided.

TIP 61: ESTABLISH A REGULAR SLEEP AND WAKE SCHEDULE

Having a regular schedule for sleeping and waking up is crucial for regulating your body's biological clock and improving sleep quality. Try to go to bed and wake up at approximately the same time every day, including on weekends, to help establish a consistent sleep rhythm. This helps your body synchronize its sleep and wake cycles, promoting a sense of regularity and predictability that can enhance the quality of your sleep over time. Additionally, maintaining a regular sleep schedule can help improve sleep efficiency by reducing the time it takes to fall asleep and minimizing interruptions during the night. By making sleep a priority and establishing a consistent sleep and wake routine, you are creating the ideal conditions for a restful night's sleep and greater productivity during the day.

TIP 62: CREATE A SLEEP-FRIENDLY ENVIRONMENT, DARK, COOL, AND QUIET

An appropriate environment is essential for promoting quality sleep. Ensure that your bedroom is dark, cool, and quiet to create the ideal conditions for sleep. This means blocking out external light with dark curtains or blinds and avoiding exposure to bright screens before bedtime, as the blue light emitted by electronic devices can interfere with natural sleep rhythms. Keep the room temperature comfortable, typically between 18°C and 22°C, to prevent heat or cold from disrupting your sleep. Additionally, minimize noise as much as possible by using earplugs or white noise machines, if necessary, to minimize disruptions during the night. By creating a sleep-friendly environment, you are setting the stage for a night of deep and restorative rest, which can enhance your productivity and well-being during the day.

TIP 63: AVOID CAFFEINE AND HEAVY MEALS BEFORE BEDTIME

Avoiding caffeine and heavy meals a few hours before bedtime can help ensure that your body is ready to relax and fall asleep. Caffeine, found in coffee, tea, sodas, and chocolate, is a stimulant that can interfere with sleep patterns, keeping you awake longer and reducing sleep quality. Additionally, heavy, fatty, or spicy foods can cause gastric discomfort and indigestion, making it difficult to relax and contributing to sleep disturbances. Therefore, it is recommended to avoid consuming these foods and beverages a few hours before bedtime to promote peaceful and restful sleep.

TIP 64: LIMIT EXPOSURE TO BLUE LIGHT FROM ELECTRONIC DEVICES BEFORE BEDTIME

The blue light emitted by electronic devices such as smartphones, tablets, computers, and TVs can suppress the production of melatonin, a hormone that regulates the sleep-wake cycle. This can interfere with the body's ability to naturally fall asleep and impair sleep quality. Therefore, it is advisable to limit exposure to blue light a few hours before bedtime. You can do this by reducing the brightness of screens, activating night mode, or using blue light-blocking glasses. Additionally, it is recommended to avoid using electronic devices in bed and replace them with relaxing activities such as reading, meditation, or gentle stretching to help prepare the body and mind for sleep.

TIP 65: PRACTICE RELAXATION TECHNIQUES BEFORE BED, SUCH AS MEDITATION OR GENTLE STRETCHING

Practicing relaxation techniques before bed can help calm the mind and body, preparing you for a restful night's sleep. Meditation, for example, can help reduce stress and anxiety, promoting a sense of calm and tranquility. You can practice meditation by focusing on your breath, visualizing peaceful imagery, or repeating relaxing mantras. Additionally, gentle stretching can help relax tense muscles and relieve accumulated tension throughout the day. Try doing some gentle yoga poses or practicing stretching techniques before bed to relax the body and mind and prepare for a rejuvenating night's sleep.

TIP 66: MAINTAIN A REGULAR EXERCISE ROUTINE

Regular physical exercise can help improve sleep quality by promoting relaxation and reducing stress. Aerobic exercises such as walking, running, swimming, or cycling can help release endorphins, neurotransmitters that promote feelings of well-being and relaxation. Additionally, strength training exercises such as weightlifting or Pilates can help reduce anxiety and promote deeper, more restorative sleep. However, it's important to avoid intense exercise close to bedtime, as this can increase energy levels and make it difficult to fall asleep. Therefore, it's recommended to maintain a regular exercise routine, preferably during the day or early afternoon, to reap the benefits of a more peaceful and revitalizing sleep.

TIP 67: AVOID LONG NAPS DURING THE DAY

While short naps during the day can be beneficial for recharging and increasing alertness, long or late naps can interfere with nighttime sleep patterns and impair sleep quality. Prolonged naps can reduce sleep pressure, making it harder to fall asleep at night and decreasing the total amount of sleep needed. Additionally, long naps can disrupt the natural sleep-wake cycle and lead to daytime drowsiness. Therefore, it's recommended to avoid long naps, especially late in the afternoon or evening, to ensure restful and quality sleep at night.

TIP 68: SET ASIDE TIME TO DISCONNECT AND RELAX BEFORE BED

Setting aside time to disconnect and relax before bed can help prepare the body and mind for a peaceful and restorative night's sleep. Turning off electronic devices such as smartphones, tablets, and computers at least an hour before bedtime can help reduce exposure to blue light and promote the production of melatonin, a hormone that regulates sleep. Additionally, practicing relaxation techniques such as meditation, deep breathing, or gentle stretching can help calm the mind and body, relieve stress, and promote deeper and more restful sleep. Therefore, it's recommended to set aside time every night to disconnect and relax before bed, creating a sleep-friendly environment and improving the quality of nighttime rest.

TIP 69: KEEP A WORRY JOURNAL TO RELEASE THOUGHTS BEFORE BED

Keeping a worry journal can be an effective strategy for releasing thoughts and concerns before bed, helping to calm the mind and promote a more peaceful sleep. Set aside a few minutes every night to write about your worries, anxieties, or restless thoughts from the day. Write freely, without worrying about grammar or cohesion, just letting your thoughts flow onto the paper. By externalizing your worries, you may feel a sense of relief and clarity, allowing your mind to relax and prepare for sleep. Additionally, keeping a worry journal can help identify recurring thought patterns and develop effective strategies for coping with stress and anxiety over time.

TIP 70: AVOID ALCOHOLIC BEVERAGES BEFORE BED

While alcohol may initially help relax and fall asleep more easily, it can interfere with sleep patterns and reduce the quality of nighttime rest. Consuming alcoholic beverages before bed can disrupt the natural sleep-wake cycle, resulting in fragmented and shallow sleep. Additionally, alcohol can suppress the production of melatonin, the sleep hormone, and increase the frequency of awakenings during the night. Therefore, it's recommended to avoid consuming alcoholic beverages in the hours leading up to bedtime, opting for healthier alternatives such as herbal tea or warm milk to promote a more peaceful and restorative sleep.

TIP 71: TRY DEEP BREATHING TECHNIQUES TO RELAX YOUR BODY AND MIND

Deep breathing techniques can be an effective tool for relaxing the body and mind, reducing stress, and promoting a calmer, more restful sleep. Set aside a few minutes before bedtime to practice deep breathing, sitting or lying comfortably in a quiet environment. Inhale deeply through your nose, filling your lungs with air, and exhale slowly through your mouth, releasing any tension or worry. Focus on the sensation of the breath entering and leaving your body, allowing your mind to calm and quieten. Repeat this breathing pattern several times, letting yourself be guided by the natural rhythm of your own breath. Experiment with different breathing techniques, such as abdominal breathing or alternate nostril breathing, to find the one that best suits your needs and preferences.

TIP 72: INVEST IN A COMFORTABLE MATTRESS AND PILLOWS

A comfortable mattress and pillows are essential for a good night's sleep. Investing in a quality mattress that provides proper support for your posture and sleep preferences can help reduce back pain and improve the quality of your rest. Likewise, choosing pillows that comfortably cradle your head and neck can help prevent aches and discomfort during the night. Look for materials and technologies that provide comfort and durability, taking into account your personal preferences for firmness and support. By investing in a quality mattress and pillows, you'll create an environment conducive to a peaceful and restorative night's sleep.

TIP 73: KEEP THE BEDROOM CLEAN AND ORGANIZED TO PROMOTE A SENSE OF CALM

A clean and organized environment can have a significant impact on the quality of your sleep. Keeping the bedroom clean and free of clutter can promote a sense of calm and tranquility, helping the mind to relax before bedtime. Set aside a few minutes every day to make the bed, put away clothes and personal belongings, and clean surfaces and floors. Additionally, consider eliminating or reducing visual clutter in the bedroom, opting for simple and minimalist décor. By creating a clean and organized environment, you'll prepare the stage for a quieter and more rejuvenating night's sleep.

TIP 74: AVOID STIMULATING ACTIVITIES BEFORE BED, SUCH AS WATCHING SUSPENSEFUL MOVIES

Stimulating activities before bed, such as watching suspenseful movies or engaging in mentally demanding tasks, can make it difficult to relax and interfere with the quality of your sleep. Exciting or stressful stimuli can increase brain activity and make it harder to fall asleep and stay asleep throughout the night. Therefore, avoid activities that may leave you feeling agitated or anxious in the hours leading up to bedtime. Instead, opt for more relaxing and calming activities such as reading a book, listening to soft music, or practicing relaxation techniques. By reducing stimulation before bed, you'll prepare your body and mind for a more serene and restful night's sleep.

TIP 75: PRACTICE SLEEP HYGIENE, SUCH AS TAKING A WARM BATH BEFORE BED

Sleep hygiene involves a series of practices and rituals that help prepare the body and mind for a peaceful and restorative night's sleep. Taking a warm bath before bed is one of these practices that can be especially effective for promoting relaxation and inducing sleep. Hot water helps relax the muscles and relieve tension accumulated throughout the day, preparing the body for rest. Additionally, the heat from the bath raises the body's temperature, and when you step out of the bath, this temperature drop signals to the body that it's time to sleep, helping to regulate the sleep cycle. Therefore, including a warm bath in your sleep hygiene routine can be an effective way to improve the quality of your nighttime rest.

TIP 76: ESTABLISH A RELAXATION RITUAL BEFORE BED, SUCH AS READING A BOOK

Establishing a relaxation ritual before bed can help calm the mind and prepare the body for a peaceful night's sleep. Reading a book is a relaxing activity that can help reduce stress and anxiety, creating an environment conducive to sleep. Choose a light and enjoyable book, avoiding themes that may be too stimulating or exciting. Set aside a few minutes every night to read before bed, creating a consistent ritual that signals to the body that it's time to relax and prepare for sleep. In addition to being an effective relaxation method, reading can also help distract the mind from worries and intrusive thoughts, making it easier to transition to sleep.

TIP 77: LIMIT FLUID INTAKE BEFORE BED TO AVOID SLEEP INTERRUPTIONS

Limiting fluid intake before bed is important to avoid sleep interruptions caused by the need to urinate during the night. Drinking large amounts of fluids before bed can increase urine production and lead to waking up multiple times during the night to use the bathroom, which can disrupt the quality of your sleep. Therefore, avoid drinking large amounts of fluids until about two hours before bedtime. If you feel thirsty before bed, opt for smaller amounts of fluids and choose options that are not diuretic, such as water or herbal tea. By limiting fluid intake before bed, you'll help ensure a quieter and uninterrupted night's sleep.

TIP 78: MAINTAIN A REGULAR MEAL SCHEDULE TO REGULATE YOUR BIOLOGICAL CLOCK

Maintaining a regular meal schedule can help regulate your body's biological clock, which in turn can improve sleep quality. The biological clock, also known as the circadian rhythm, regulates the body's sleep and wake patterns and is influenced by various factors, including meal times. By eating at consistent times every day, you help your body establish a healthy routine, which can facilitate the transition to sleep at night. Try to keep your meal times as regular as possible, avoiding large meals late at night, which can make digestion difficult and interfere with sleep.

TIP 79: TRY PROGRESSIVE MUSCLE RELAXATION TECHNIQUES TO RELIEVE TENSION

Progressive muscle relaxation is a relaxation technique that involves systematically tensing and relaxing the muscles of the body to relieve tension and promote relaxation. Begin by focusing on one part of the body, such as the muscles of the forehead, and tense them for a few seconds before releasing the tension and fully relaxing. Then, move on to the next part of the body, such as the muscles of the cheeks, neck, shoulders, arms, and so on, until you have worked all major muscle groups. Practicing progressive muscle relaxation regularly before bed can help calm the mind and body, preparing you for a peaceful and restful night's sleep.

TIP 80: AVOID EXCITING OR STRESSFUL ACTIVITIES BEFORE BED

Avoiding exciting or stressful activities before bed is essential for preparing the body and mind for a good night's sleep. Exciting activities, such as watching suspenseful movies or discussing important issues, can stimulate the brain and increase levels of arousal, making it harder to relax and fall asleep. Similarly, stressful activities, such as solving work problems or dealing with interpersonal conflicts, can cause anxiety and worry, interfering with sleep quality. Therefore, it's important to avoid these activities in the hours before bedtime and opt for more relaxing and tranquil activities such as reading a book, listening to soft music, or practicing relaxation techniques. This will help calm the mind and prepare the body for a peaceful and restorative night's sleep.

TIP 81: USE VISUALIZATION TECHNIQUES TO INDUCE A STATE OF RELAXATION BEFORE BED

Visualization is a powerful technique for relaxing the mind and body before bed. To practice visualization, find a quiet and comfortable place to lie down. Close your eyes and begin to imagine a calm and serene place or scene, such as a quiet beach, lush forest, or field of flowers. Focus on all the sensory details of this place - the colors, sounds, smells, and tactile sensations. Allow yourself to fully immerse in this scene, allowing it to envelop you in a sense of peace and deep relaxation. Continue the visualization until you feel completely relaxed and ready to fall asleep.

TIP 82: MAKE A TO-DO LIST FOR THE NEXT DAY TO RELEASE WORRIES BEFORE BED

Making a to-do list for the next day can help release worries and anxieties that may be disrupting your sleep. Set aside a few minutes before bed to write down all the tasks you need to accomplish the following day. This will help empty your mind, transferring your concerns onto paper and allowing you to relax and prepare for a good night's sleep. Additionally, having a clear and organized to-do list for the next day can help reduce stress and increase productivity when you wake up in the morning.

TIP 83: PRACTICE GRATITUDE BEFORE BED, REFLECTING ON THE POSITIVE ASPECTS OF THE DAY

Practicing gratitude before bed can help promote a state of relaxation and contentment, which is essential for a good night's sleep. Set aside a few minutes before bedtime to reflect on the positive aspects of your day and identify things you are grateful for. This may include happy moments, personal achievements, rewarding experiences, or simply things you appreciate in your life. Focus on feelings of gratitude and appreciation, allowing them to fill your mind and heart with a sense of peace and contentment. This practice can help reduce stress and anxiety, promoting a more peaceful and restful sleep.

TIP 84: TRY LIGHT THERAPY TO REGULATE THE SLEEP CYCLE

Light therapy is a technique that uses bright lights to help regulate the sleep-wake cycle. This technique is especially useful for people who suffer from sleep disorders such as insomnia or seasonal affective disorder. Exposure to bright light, especially in the morning, can help suppress the production of melatonin, the sleep hormone, and regulate the internal biological clock. There are commercially available light therapy devices that can be used at home, and many of them offer customized options for intensity and duration to meet individual sleep needs.

TIP 85: USE A SLEEP MASK TO BLOCK LIGHT AND PROMOTE DEEPER SLEEP

A sleep mask can be a simple and effective solution for blocking excess light and promoting deeper, more restful sleep. Light can interfere with your sleep-wake cycle, especially if you're exposed to bright light sources during the night, such as streetlights or electronic devices. A comfortable and adjustable sleep mask can help block out light completely and create a dark, sleep-friendly environment. Additionally, some sleep masks also offer additional benefits, such as gel eye pads or breathable fabrics for added comfort during the night.

TIP 86: AVOID EXCESSIVE USE OF ELECTRONIC DEVICES IN BED

Excessive use of electronic devices in bed, such as smartphones, tablets, or laptops, can interfere with sleep and disrupt sleep quality. The blue light emitted by these devices can suppress the production of melatonin, the sleep hormone, and interfere with the natural sleep-wake cycle. Additionally, the stimulating or stressful content found in apps or social media can agitate the mind and make it difficult to relax before bed. To promote a calmer, more restful sleep, it's important to limit the use of electronic devices in bed and create a technology-free environment at least one hour before bedtime.

TIP 87: PRACTICE COUNTDOWN TECHNIQUE TO INDUCE SLEEP

The countdown technique is a simple and effective strategy for calming the mind and inducing sleep. When lying in bed, close your eyes and start counting down, beginning from a high number like 100, and slowly decreasing with each breath. Focus on the counting and try to visualize each number as you imagine it. This can help distract the mind from intrusive thoughts or worries and relax the body, preparing it for sleep. Keep counting until you feel drowsy and ready to fall asleep.

TIP 88: MAINTAIN A SEPARATE WORK ENVIRONMENT FROM THE BEDROOM TO ASSOCIATE THE BEDROOM SOLELY WITH SLEEP

Maintaining a separate work environment from the bedroom is important for creating a mental association between the bedroom and sleep. If possible, avoid engaging in work-related activities, such as answering emails or making phone calls, in the bedroom. Instead, reserve the bedroom exclusively for relaxing activities, such as sleeping and unwinding. This helps condition your brain to associate the bedroom with rest and relaxation, making it easier to fall asleep and improving sleep quality.

TIP 89: AVOID ARGUMENTS BEFORE BED TO MAINTAIN A CALM ENVIRONMENT

Avoiding arguments before bed is essential for maintaining a calm and sleep-friendly environment. Emotional conflicts or confrontations can stimulate the mind and increase stress levels, making it harder to relax and fall asleep. Try to resolve any disagreements or conflicts during the day and reserve the time before bed for relaxing and peaceful activities, such as reading a book or practicing relaxation techniques. This helps promote a calm and serene environment, setting the stage for a restful and revitalizing night's sleep.

TIP 90: PRACTICE GENTLE YOGA BEFORE BED TO RELAX THE BODY AND MIND

Practicing gentle yoga before bed can be an effective way to relax the body and mind, preparing for a good night's sleep. Gentle yoga poses help release accumulated muscle tension throughout the day and calm the nervous system, promoting a deep sense of relaxation. Additionally, mindful breathing and gentle movements help calm the mind, reducing stress and anxiety levels. Try incorporating some simple yoga poses, such as Happy Baby pose or Cat-Cow pose, into your nighttime routine to promote a quieter and more restorative sleep.

Tip 91: Try aromatherapy with relaxing essential oils, like lavender.

Aromatherapy is a technique that uses aromatic essential oils to promote physical and emotional well-being. Lavender essential oil is known for its relaxing and calming properties, making it a popular choice for promoting sleep. Try adding a few drops of lavender essential oil to an aromatherapy diffuser before bedtime or apply it gently to your wrists and the back of your neck. The soft and comforting aroma of lavender can help reduce stress and anxiety, inducing a state of deep relaxation and facilitating sleep.

Tip 92: Use self-guided relaxation techniques, such as imagining a peaceful location.

Self-guided relaxation techniques are an effective way to calm the mind and relax the body before sleep. A simple and effective technique is to imagine a peaceful and serene location where you feel calm and safe. Close your eyes and begin visualizing your tranquil location, paying attention to details like colors, sounds, and smells. Focus on images that evoke feelings of peace and serenity, such as a quiet beach at sunset or a lush garden on a spring afternoon. As you concentrate on your visualization, allow yourself to relax completely, releasing any tension or worry. This technique can help calm the restless mind and prepare you for a peaceful and restful night's sleep.

TIP 93: AVOID VIGOROUS EXERCISE BEFORE BEDTIME.

While regular exercise is beneficial for sleep quality, it's important to avoid vigorous exercise before bedtime. Vigorous exercise can increase heart rate and body temperature, which can make it difficult to transition to sleep. Instead, opt for gentler and relaxing activities in the evening, such as gentle yoga or leisurely walks. This will help calm the body and mind, preparing you for a peaceful night's sleep.

Tip 94: Try acupressure techniques to relieve tension before sleep.

Acupressure is a technique based on traditional Chinese medicine that involves applying pressure to specific points on the body to relieve tension and promote relaxation. Try applying gentle pressure to points such as the HT7 acupressure point, located on the inside of the wrist between the wrist tendons. Pressing this point can help calm the mind and relieve anxiety, facilitating sleep. Other acupressure points that may be helpful for promoting sleep include the Yintang point, located between the eyebrows, and the KD3 point, located on the bottom of the foot, in the midline between the Achilles tendon and the ankle. Try these acupressure techniques before sleep to relax the body and mind and promote a peaceful night's sleep.

Tip 95: Maintain a regular sleep pattern, even on weekends.

Maintaining a regular sleep pattern, going to bed and waking up at roughly the same time every day, is essential for regulating the biological clock and improving sleep quality. Even on weekends, try to maintain your sleep schedule to avoid disruptions in the sleep-wake cycle. While it may be tempting to sleep in later on weekends, this can disrupt your biological clock and make it difficult to adjust during the week. Therefore, try to maintain a regular sleep schedule, even on days off, to ensure restorative sleep and a greater sense of well-being over time.

Tip 96: Avoid late afternoon naps to avoid interfering with nighttime sleep.

While a short nap during the day can be refreshing, napping late in the afternoon can interfere with nighttime sleep. It's best to avoid naps after 3 p.m., as this can impair your ability to fall asleep at night and compromise sleep quality. If you feel the need to rest during the day, opt for short naps of 20 to 30 minutes and avoid extending sleep time in the afternoon to ensure it doesn't affect your nighttime sleep.

Tip 97: Try relaxing music or nature sounds to promote sleep.

Relaxing music and nature sounds can be effective tools for inducing sleep and improving the quality of rest. Try listening to gentle music, such as classical music, jazz, or ambient music, before bed to calm the mind and relax the body. Additionally, nature sounds, such as the sound of rain, ocean waves, or bird song, can create a tranquil environment conducive to sleep. Use comfortable headphones or an audio playback device with low volume to enjoy these relaxing sounds as you prepare for sleep.

Tip 98: Use a tension release technique, such as squeezing and relaxing muscles, before sleep.

Before lying down, try a tension release technique to relax the body and mind. A simple and effective technique is to squeeze and relax the muscles progressively, starting from the feet and working up to the head. As you lie comfortably in bed, contract the muscles in your feet and hold the tension for a few seconds before releasing them completely. Then, repeat the process with the muscles in your legs, abdomen, arms, face, and neck, focusing on releasing any accumulated tension. This progressive muscle relaxation technique can help relieve stress and prepare the body for a peaceful and restful night's sleep.

Tip 99: Practice the "quiet mind" technique to calm the mind before sleep.

Before sleep, practice the "quiet mind" technique to calm your thoughts and prepare for a peaceful night's sleep. Find a comfortable place to sit or lie down, close your eyes, and focus on your breathing. As you inhale and exhale, observe the thoughts that arise in your mind without attaching to them. Imagine each thought as a cloud passing through the sky of your consciousness, allowing them to dissipate naturally. Focus on the feeling of relaxation that arises as your mind becomes quieter and more serene. This simple practice can help calm the restless mind and promote a more restful sleep.

Tip 100: Consult a healthcare professional if you have persistent sleep problems.

If you're experiencing persistent sleep problems, it's important to consult a healthcare professional for proper evaluation and guidance. A doctor or sleep specialist can help identify the underlying causes of your sleep disorder and recommend a personalized treatment plan. This may include lifestyle changes, behavioral therapy, medications, or other interventions, depending on the nature and severity of your sleep problem. Don't hesitate to seek help if you're experiencing difficulty sleeping, as a good night's sleep is essential for overall health and well-being.

Throughout this topic, we've explored a wide range of tips and strategies for improving sleep quality and increasing productivity. From establishing a regular sleep schedule to practicing relaxation techniques before bed, each suggestion is designed to help you create an environment conducive to restorative and revitalizing sleep.

Quality sleep plays a fundamental role in our physical, mental, and emotional health, affecting our ability to concentrate, make decisions, and perform overall. By implementing these tips into your daily routine, you can promote healthy sleep habits that will improve your quality of life and increase your effectiveness during the day.

However, it's important to recognize that each person is unique, and not all strategies will work the same way for everyone. Experiment with different approaches and adapt them according to your individual needs and preferences. And remember, if you're experiencing persistent sleep difficulties, don't hesitate to seek professional guidance from a doctor or sleep specialist.

By prioritizing quality sleep and adopting practices that promote adequate rest, you'll be investing in your long-term health and well-being, empowering yourself to face each day with energy, mental clarity, and productivity.

TIP 101: CULTIVATE FAITH AND SPIRITUALITY

Regardless of your specific religious belief, cultivating faith and spirituality can be a powerful resource for finding inner peace and facing life's challenges with courage and hope. Take time to connect with your spirituality, whether through prayer, meditation, reading sacred texts, or participating in religious communities. Find comfort and inspiration in your faith, allowing it to illuminate your path and strengthen your resilience in the face of adversity.

Faith and spirituality have the power to nurture our soul, offering comfort in times of difficulty and guidance in times of uncertainty. They remind us that we are not alone in our journeys but connected to something greater than ourselves. By cultivating faith, we find a source of hope that transcends external circumstances and sustains us in the most challenging moments.

Furthermore, the practice of spirituality often encourages us to cultivate virtues such as compassion, forgiveness, and gratitude, which are essential for fostering healthy relationships, managing stress, and finding meaning in our lives. By integrating faith into our daily routine, we nurture not only our spiritual health but also our mental, emotional, and physical health.

Regardless of individual beliefs, faith and spirituality offer a refuge of peace and a sense of purpose that can deeply enrich our lives. By taking time to cultivate this essential dimension of our being, we open the doors to greater serenity, gratitude, and connection to something beyond ourselves. May faith guide us on our journeys, strengthening and inspiring us to live with integrity, compassion, and hope.

Final Thoughts

In this journey of self-improvement and well-being, we've explored a wide range of tips, practices, and insights aimed at nurturing not only our body but also our mind and spirit. From adopting healthy eating and exercise habits to cultivating inner peace, resilience, and spirituality, every page of this book is designed to inspire and empower you to live a full and meaningful life.

Throughout these pages, you've discovered ways to enhance your physical, emotional, and spiritual health, recognizing the importance of caring for yourself holistically. You've learned to nourish your body with nutritious foods, strengthen your mind with relaxation practices, and feed your soul with gratitude, compassion, and purpose.

Remember that the path to well-being is not a linear journey. There will be ups and downs, challenges and triumphs, but every step you take toward self-awareness and self-development is a victory in itself. Allow yourself to be kind to yourself during this process, recognizing that progress comes with time and consistent practice.

May this book be an inspiring guide on your journey of personal growth, and may the lessons learned here accompany you in all aspects of your life. May you find joy in the journey, strength in adversity, and gratitude in every moment. May you live with authenticity, purpose, and wholeness, radiating love and light to the world around you.

May this book be the beginning of an exciting new adventure in pursuit of a healthier, more meaningful, and fulfilling life. The power is in your hands to create the life you desire. May you move forward with courage, determination, and a heart full of hope.

May your journey be abundant in blessings, achievements, and moments of profound happiness. And may you always remember the incredible potential that resides within you, waiting to be awakened and manifested to the world.

May you live each day with gratitude, purpose, and joy, making the world a better place simply by being yourself. Thank you for embarking on this journey with us. May your life be a continuous celebration of the miracle of being human.

With love and gratitude,

F. H. RODRIGUES